DOG
Training Smackdown
The A-Z on Puppy & Dog Training

MICAH JACK

Dog Training Smackdown

The A - Z of Puppy & Dog Training

Micah Jack

Copyright © 2019 Micah Jack

ISBN: 978-1-63750-194-8

Table of Contents

Introduction

Getting a new puppy or dog is usually an exciting thing for any family. There is a good reason why dogs are referred to as men's best friend, and a devoted dog is more than just a pet, it's a treasured member of the family. To reach that stage of affection and companionship, it is far crucial to begin your puppy or dog off on the right foot of training.

A strong training in obedience and good manners is vital to making your dog, and you, happier and healthier.

How does your dog sit when you tell it to and mine doesn't?

How can your dog respond to you like that?

"Wow! It comes when you tell it to" - *sounds familiar?* If it does, you need to make investments into a little bit of primary dog schooling. Start teaching your dog from a younger age because the first few months of its life is when you have the best influence on it; that is when it is formed into the dog it becomes when it's all grown up.

The most essential dog education is to get your dog to take a seat and remain calm. Teaching it those commands are crucial for it to get adjusted to. Those instructions are used for numerous unique reasons, if you are in a competition and your dog jumps up and you are unable to make it sit still, this will definitely get him off the competition. To "*come*" is the most primary command.

If you take your dog for a walk and you allow it off the leash, you expect it to return back to you and not run around the park with you chasing after it, shouting for it to *"get here right this instant"*. That could be downright embarrassing!

To train your dog the right way to act requires the maximum fundamental techniques; however continuity is essential in its traning. The simplest way to get it to come back is to have a toy on one hand and a treat on the other.

When you are in a residential area, stroll a few paces away from it, keep out the toy and call it to you excitingly, when it comes over; supply it a treat, always use the command for come during the duration of the training. Doing this numerous times a day is an exceptional way to educate it, but remember to take lengthy breaks so it doesn't get bored and stop taking part in it, and don't overlook the treats!

Getting it to sit down could be more difficult but again this technnique requires fundamental dog schooling. If you have mastered the *"come"* *command*, call it to you, place your hand at the tip of its back and say *"take a seat"* at the same time lightly push it down on its backside, while it places its bottom down, deliver it a treat and a number of praises.

In case you want it to sit down longer, just put off giving it the treat and the reward, get it to sit, however take your time bending all the way down to it and feeding it its treat.

Basic dog education is straightforward and very powerful. It needs to also be an exciting experience for you and your dog; it shouldn't be an hourly affair daily, merely 5 minutes or so. Don't overlook rewarding your dog and yourself for all the "hard" work!

Permit me to start with simple dog and puppy training as you read further, inorder to have the dog or puppy a new domestic addition to the house members list as much as making sure it is well socialized and behaved.

My coaching program rescues an undesirable, untrained, "unadoptable" guard dog. This publication shows my puppy/dog natural pet coaching program for changing any dog or puppy from spoiled purebred pup to shelter-shocked rescue which becomes a friendly companion in under 14 days or less. Within a several days array, these puppies experience a fantastic transformation because they know to trust my own methodology including my 6 basic commands, and conquer their behaviour difficulties, finally becoming well-mannered pets as well as support dogs by producing perfect obedience from day one through principles, bounds, along with also calm-assertive leadership. This lesson unites each dog having a forever family. As a vetenary physician, I've shared the wisdom gained from working with various dogs of diverse breed and character to help individuals develop their own pets to well-trained dog that will cause you to feel great about instruction and rewarding your pet with wellness organic dog treats.

This training starts with the fundamentals establishing focus, control and building confidence (trust), and mastering training techniques. Therein, I explain the 6 common commands i teach every dog: *HEEL, NO, SIT, STAY, DOWN, and OFF* commands. Furthermore; you will explicitly learn solutions to common canine behavior problems, how to avoid the most common mistakes dog/puppy owners make raising puppies and young dogs, housetraining and house training issues, how to correct any issue before it becomes a problem such as: potty training (*perfect for potty training which gives your puppy the best chance for success when it comes to potty training*), door dashing, handling biting, leash pulling, jumping up, barking, aggression, chewing, and other behavioral issues, common mealtime misbehaviors and unique exercises and play to bring out the best in every breed.

This book is packed with everything you need to

know to raise and care for your dog, this book will

help you communicate and bond with one another

in a way that makes training easier, more

rewarding, and—most of all—fun. Likewise

includes easy-to-follow steps, illustrative examples,

tried-and-true tips and tricks.

CHAPTER 1

Educating your New Puppy or Dog

Bringing a new domestic dog into the family is continually an interesting and fun experience. Absolutely everyone wants to play with, cuddle and maintain the little ball of fur. The major thought on the minds of most new puppy owners is training the new addition to the family; however it's very important that puppy education and socialization begins as early as possible.

In a few ways; training a puppy is simpler than educating an adult or adolescent dog.

One reason is that the domestic dog is essentially a *"blank slate"*. However, the puppy may be easier to educate than an older dog.

One problem in educating a new puppy is that they are very easily prone to distraction than adolescent and adult dogs. The whole world is new to a puppy, and every new experience creates a new risk and a distraction. For that reason, it's far excellent to keep schooling sessions brief when running with a puppy, and to maintain each schooling classes on a high quality level.

Socializing a brand new puppy is a vital part of any education program and it's very crucial for socialization to start early. The window for socialization is very quick, and a dog that isn't always well socialized to human beings, puppies and other animals especially when it is four months old, by no means develops the socialization it wishes to adopt and end up a terrific dog.

Socialization training is critical to making your new puppy an awesome dog, as dog aggression is a developing problem in many areas. A well socialized dog learns a way to play properly with different puppies, and overly aggressive play is punished by the other puppies in the play region.

This sort of play mastering is something that takes place amongst siblings in litters of puppies. As the dogs play with each other, they learn what's appropriate and what isn't.

Inappropriate behavior, consisting of tough biting or scratching, is punished by the other dogs, through the mother dog, or both.

Unfortunately, many puppies are eliminated from their mothers and bought or adopted before this socialization has completely come about. Consequently, puppy play classes are a completely important part of any puppy schooling education. Most top domestic dog preschool training programs provide time in every session for this type of dog interplay.

Introducing your puppy to new experiences and

new places is also an essential part of dog education. Teaching your dog to be obedient and responsive, even in the face of many distractions, is very crucial when educating dogs and puppies.

One wonderful technique to socialise your domestic dog to new humans and new dogs is to take it on a ride to your nearby pet shop and these stores may be incredible places for puppies to get used to new sights, sounds and smells. Of course you will want to ensure the shop permits pets earlier than heading over.

Getting to know the way to interact with other puppies is some thing that generally would arise between littermates. But, since most dogs are removed from their mothers so soon, this littermate socialization often does not finish properly.

One important lesson puppies learn from their littermates and from the mother dog is a way to chunk, and how not to chew for longer periods. Dogs certainly play differently, and their thick pores and skin protects them from most bites. But, when one pup bites too rough, the other puppies, or the mom dog, quickly reprimand it, often by way of keeping hold on the scruff of its neck until it submits.

The high-quality way to socialise your dog is to

have it play with multitudes of other dogs. It's also exceptional for the domestic dog to play with a few pet dogs, as long as they're friendly and properly socialized. Many groups have domestic dog playschool and doggy kindergarten

Lessons to Learn:

These instructions can be a terrific way to socialize any domestic dog, and for the handler and domestic dog alike to learn a few fundamental obedience capabilities. Whilst socializing puppies, it's highly satisfactory to let them play on their own and work out their personal troubles when it comes to seemly rough play. The simplest time the proprietors need to step in is if one dog is hurting every other, or if a severe fight breaks out. Other than that, the proprietors ought to genuinely stand by and watch the dogs interact.

Even as this socialization is taking place, the percentage hierarchy usually turns out to be apparent. Some dogs are ultra-submissive, rolling on their backs and baring their teeths at the slightest provocation. Different puppies inside the class can be dominant, ordering the other puppies around and telling them what to do. Observing the dogs play, and figuring out what sort of character trends your domestic dog has, can be very valuable in determining the best way to continue with greater superior schooling.

As the socialization method proceeds, of course, it will be essential to introduce the dogs to all forms of human beings in addition to all types of puppies. Luckily, the domestic dog kindergarten style makes this system pretty smooth, because each dog gets to interact with every human. It's very crucial that the domestic dog be exposed to guys, and ladies, antique (old) humans and youngsters, black humans and white people. Dogs do not see each human as the identical. To a dog, a man and a lady are completely different animals.

It's also crucial to introduce the pup to a spread of other animals, especially in a multi pet family.

Introducing the dog to pleasant cat is crucial as with introductions to different animals. The dog may additionally encounter rabbits, guinea pigs and so on. In case your household consists of a more uncommon creature, it's highly crucial to introduce the pup to it as early as possible, however to do it in a way that is safe for both animals.

It is often fine to start by introducing the domestic dog to the odor of the other animal. This may be achieved easily by setting a chunk of the animals bedding, like a towel or mattress liner, near where the puppy/dog sleeps. As soon as the dog is conversant to the scent of the other creature, it is much more likely to accept the animal as just every other family member.

It is very crucial for dog owners to structure their puppy's surroundings in order that the domestic dog is rewarded for suitable behaviors and not rewarded for others. One true example of this is jumping on human beings.

Many human beings inadvertently praise this conduct because it seems cute. Even if it's likely that jumping may be cute for a ten pound pup, it's not going to be so adorable while that domestic dog has grown into a one hundred pound dog. Rather than praise the dog for jumping, attempt rewarding it for sitting as a substitute. This form of advantageous reinforcement will bring about a well behaved adult dog that could be a valued member of the family and the community at large.

This type of reinforcement can also be utilized in educating the brand new puppy. For example, teaching a puppy to use a completely unique floor including gravel or asphalt is a great method. The idea is that the dog will master this floor and therefore be reluctant to use other surfaces (like your kitchen carpet for instance) as a potty.

It's always first-class to introduce a new puppy or dog to the household especially when the family is calm and stable. This is why animal care specialists discourage mother and father from giving dogs and kittens as holiday presents. The holiday season is usually too busy, with far too many distractions, for a young puppy or kitten to get the eye it deserves. It is nice to wait till the vacations have passed rather than introducing the new member of the family.

Once the puppy is part of the family, there are few matters it must be able to examine. One of the first demanding situations of a domestic dog could be mastering to climb up and down the stairs. Many dogs are afraid of stairs, and that usually means that they do not understand the way to climb them well. It's very critical for the dog's owner to slowly build the self assurance of the dog, taking off at the bottom of the steps. In otherwords, a wide stairway will possibly be much less frightening to the doggy.

To build confidence, the owner should go up a step, and then encourage the dog to join them, using their voice, treats or a toy. After the dog has joined you on the first stair, go back down and repeat the method till the puppy will move up that step on its own. It is essential to build confidence slowly and not to rush the process. Taking it one step at a time is a great way to train the puppy to not be frightened of stairs.

Some other things every new puppy needs to examine is the way to accept the collar. Gaining knowledge on wearing a collar is vital to every dog, however many puppies are baffled, apprehensive and bewildered via this new piece of gadget. Many puppies continuously try and do away with their new collar through pawing and pulling at it.

Such is vital while choosing a collar on your new domestic dog. A nicely fitted collar, chosen for your puppy's length, is much more likely to be cozy and regular. At the same time a choke, slip and schooling collar may be proper training aids, they must by no means be used alternatively for a sturdy buckle type collar. And of course that collar should have an identity tag and license connected. This identification can be essential in having your puppy again if it becomes separated from you.

The quality and manner to introduce the puppy to the collar is to actually place the collar on and permit it to squirm, leap, roll and paw at the shade to its heart's content material. It's very important to not encourage this conduct with the aid of seeking to soothe the puppy, however it's also just as important not to punish or reprimand the dog.

The high-quality approach is to forget about the puppy and its probable struggle with the collar on. Introducing distractions, including food, toys or playing, is a superb way to get the domestic dog used to the collar. Getting the puppy to play, devour and drink at the same time as wearing the collar is an extraordinary way to get it used to it. After a few days, most dogs will not even remember they are wearing a collar.

CHAPTER 2

How to Teach Your Puppy/Dog Proper Socialization Knowledge

Teaching a puppy or a dog the right socialization skills is important for the safety of both your dog and other dogs with which it comes in contact. A properly socialized dog is a happy dog, and a pleasure to be around for both human beings and animals. A poorly socialized dog or one without socialization knowledge in any respect is a threat to different animals, other humans or even its own family.

Socialization is easily achieved when the puppy is young and it's very important to remember that the socialization knowledge the puppy learns will have an effect on its conduct for the duration of its life.

A dog that is nicely socialized may neither be fearful nor competitive towards other animals or people. A nicely socialized dog will revel in every new experience and take it in good strides rather than being fearful or competitive.

Puppies that aren't properly socialized often attack because of fear, and such a dog can turn out to be a risk and a liability to the family who owns it. Improperly socialized puppies are also not able to conform to new situations. A recurring activity like a journey to the vets or to a pal's residence can speedily strain the dog out and result in all forms of issues.

Socialization is nicely accomplished while the puppy is very young, perhaps around 12 weeks of age. Even after 12 weeks, however, it's always crucial that the puppy continues its socialization which will refine its all-important social abilties. It's far viable to socialize an older puppy, but it's very tough to gain grounds after the all-essential 12 week period has passed.

There are **do's** and **dont's** when it comes to properly socializing any puppy.

Allow me to start with what to do. Later in this book, we will explore what to keep away from.

Puppy/Dog Socialization Do's

- Make all the socialization activities as nice and non-threatening for the puppy as possible. If a pup's first enjoyable experience with any new encounter is an unappealing one, it is going to be very hard to undo that in the dog's thoughts. In some cases, an early trauma can morph into a phobia that can close for an entire life. It's far better to take matters gradually and keep away from having the dog to become fearful.

- Strive to invite your pals over to satisfy the brand new domestic dog. It's always crucial to encourage a specific human interaction and relationship in the puppy's circle of acquaintances, inclusive of men, ladies, youngsters, adults, as well as humans of many numerous ethnic backgrounds and ages.

- Also invite pleasant and healthy dogs over to satisfy your puppy. It's very important for the puppy to interact with a huge variety of different animals, which includes cats, hamsters, rabbits and other animals it is prone to meet. It's also crucial to make certain that each animal the puppy comes in contact with, have acquired all important vaccinations.

- Take the dog to many special locations, along

with purchasing centers, pet stores, parks, college playgrounds and on walks across the community. Strive to show the puppy places where there will be crowds of people and plenty of diverse interest taking place.

- Take the domestic dog for brief rides in the automobile. At some stage in these rides, make certain to slow the car from time to time and let the puppy look out the window.

- Introduce your dog to a selection of gadgets that can be unfamiliar. The puppy needs to be exposed to unusual gadgets like bags, bins, vacuum cleaners, umbrellas, hats, and many others that may be scary to him. Allow and inspire the dog to discover these gadgets and see that he has nothing to fear from them.

- Get the dog used to a spread of objects by rearranging familiar ones. Truely putting a chair the other way up, or placing a table on its facet, creates an item that your domestic dog will perceive as absolutely new.

- Get the puppy used to unusual techniques like being brushed, bathed, having the nails clipped, enamel cleaned, ears wiped clean, etc. Your groomer and your veterinarian with assist with this.

- Introduce the puppy to common matters

across the house, inclusive of stairs. Additionally introduce the domestic dog to the collar and leash, so it may be comfy with these objects.

Puppy/Dog Socialization Don'ts

There are some matters to keep away from when socializing a dog.

These socialization dont's, are:

- Do not abandon the domestic dog on the ground. An assault, or maybe a surprise inspection, through an unknown animal may want to traumatize the domestic dog and hurt its socialization.

- Do not involuntarily praise primarily fear

based conduct. When the puppy indicates fear, it is normal to try and sooth it, but this could encourage the fear based conduct and make it worse. On account that biting is mostly a fear based totally conduct, reinforcing fear can create problems with biting.

- Do not pressurize or rush the socialization system. It is essential to allow the dog to socialize at its personal tempo.

- Do not try to do too much too soon. Young dogs have quick attention spans, and pressing with instructions after that attention span has surpassed may be a waste of your time and your puppy.

- Do not wait too long to begin. There may be a short window in which to start the socialization system. A young domestic dog is a blank slate, and it is critical to fill that slate with wonderful socialization competencies as early as possible.

CHAPTER 3

Dogs' Fundamental Commands

There are of course many reasons for dog owners to want a relaxed, obedient and devoted dog. For one reason, obedient and trained puppies are happier puppies, far less in all likelihood to get into tussles with people or with other dogs.

Another reason is that most neighbourhoods require that dogs residing in their environs be well trained. That is specifically true because lots of breeds tend to have aggressive and behaviorial troubles especially breeds like *pit bulls* and *rottweilers* for instance.

Training your dog nicely will also make it a great member of the family, especially in households in which there are younger kids. Many researches have proven that proper dog training makes a massive effect when it comes to cutting down the wide variety of dog bites and other behaviorial problems encountered by dog owning households.

While thinking about training your personal dog, or having a personal trainer assist you in teaching it, there are certain fundamental instructions that should be mastered for a dog to be fully trained.

Those simple instructions include:

- **Heel** - It's very important for dogs to stroll

beside its owner on a free lead, neither pulling beforehand nor lagging behind.

- **Response to the word "No"** - The phrase "NO" is one word that every dog must understand. Teaching your dog to respond to this essential word can save you a ton of hassles.

- **Sit down** - Training your dog to sit down on command is a vital part of any dog training application.

- **Stay** - A well trained dog must remain wherein his or her proprietor commands, so; **"stay"** is an essential command in dog training.

- **Down** - Lying down on command is more

than just an adorable trick; it's basically a key thing in any dog training program.

The simple obedience commands that each dog have to understand are *"heel"*, "come", *"no"*, *"sit"*, *"stay"*, *"down" and "off"*. These six commands shape the foundation of every fundamental obedience education and it is essential that you and your dog grasp these fundamental commands. These are the fundamentals, and it is going to be difficult to convey into different instructions, or to correct problematic behaviors, without having mastered the basics.

We shall hereby discuss each command sequentially.

The Heel Command

Always begin with the most basic command of all, *the "heel" command.* Teaching a dog to heel is essentially the first step in coaching the dog to stroll nicely while on the leash. The proper region for the dog to stroll is at your side, neither lagging at the back nor straining to get ahead.

If your dog begins to forge beforehand on the lead, gently tug on the leash. For the purpose of training, this will tighten the collar and provide the dog a gentle reminder to fall back in line. If the dog starts to lag at the back, lightly urge him forward. A lure or toy is a great tool for the dog that constantly lags behind.

Once the dog is continuously strolling at your side, try to increase your tempo and encourage the dog to match hits tempo with yours. It must continually be the dog who adjusts his tempo to you; you have to in no way alter your pace to fulfill the wishes of the dog.

The Word "NO"

The phrase *"No"* is a vital one for your dog to analyze, and one that will be useful if you must continue in your dog training. It is crucial that the dog learn to reply to a pointy *"no"* right away and obediently.

The "Sit" Command

The *"take a seat command"* is another crucial training in dog schooling. Teaching a dog to sit down on command, the use of voice instructions alone, will shape the foundation of its schooling, so it's far crucial for the dog to master this vital talent.

The *sit down command* may be mixed with the *heel command*. As you walk alongside your dog, stop all of a sudden. If your dog does not stop when you do, apply a sharp tug on the leash to remind the dog.

Many puppies will instinctively stop when you do, even as others need to be reminded by using **the** *leash and the training collar.*

Once the dog has stopped at your side, urge him to take a seat by pushing gently on his hindquarters. It's very vital not to use an excessive amount of pressure, or to push it down. Doing so may want to frighten, or maybe injure the dog.

Alternatively, follow a consistent downward strain. Most dogs will understand this as a *take a seat command*. It's far essential to mention the word sit as you do that.

Repeat this process occasionally by means of *strolling, stopping and sitting your dog*. After a few repetitions, the dog will probably begin to take a seat position on its own each time it stops. It's far

vital to mention the word sit down in order for the

dog to learn to respond to voice instructions in the

long run.

The "Stay" Command

Like the *sit down command*, **the stay command** is an

essential and more advanced training. For instance,

the stay command is central to teaching the dog to

come back which is in turn crucial to off leash

strollings.

The *stay command* may be made into an extension of

the sit down command. Have your dog taken a seat,

and even as it's sitting, slowly move back from the

dog. If the dog starts to follow you, as it's in all likelihood at first, come back to the dog and tell it to take a seat once more. Repeat this manner till you can reach the end of the leash without your dog getting up from a sitting position.

After the dog is consistently staying whenever you suggest, you can attempt dropping the leash and backing slowly away. It will probably take the dog some time to stay in a position without moving or getting distracted.

The "Down" Command

The *down command* is another crucial part of any simple dog training command. Teaching a dog to lie down on command is much more than a unique trick. The down command is very essential in regaining control of a dog, or stopping a dog who's engaged in an inappropriate behavior.

The "Off" Command

The "off command" is simply as crucial as the other instructions, and it forms the basis for future education, especially while training the dog to stop chasing humans, automobiles, bikes, cats, and so forth.

For example, while training a dog to stay while a bicycle moves away, the proprietor might stand with the dog frivolously at the leash. If the dog begins to stress towards the leash, the owner sharply voices an *"off" command* observed by means of a tug of the leash. Eventually the dog will discover ways to reply to the voice command on its own.

Dog education does tons more than simply to create an obedient, inclined partner. Educating your dog nicely certainly strengthens the bond that already exists among dogs and handler. Dogs are computer animals, and that they look to their computer chief to tell them what to do. ***The key to a successful dog education is to set you up as an absolute leader.***

Setting up yourself as a computer leader is a

completely crucial concept for any dog instructor to comprehend. There's always one leader, and the proprietor needs to set him or herself to be the dominant animal. Failure to do so results in behaviorial problems.

A well trained dog will respond well to all of the owner's instructions, and will no longer show tension, displeasure or confusion. A very good dog training education recognises the importance of allowing the dog to simply do what is expected of it, and could use high quality reinforcement to reward desired behaviors.

In addition to making the dog an excellent member

of the family, submission tutoring is a first class routine to meet some of the dog's very own desires, including the need for exercising, the security that comes with knowing what's expected of it, a sense of achievement and a terrific working relationship with its handler. Dog schooling offers the dog a crucial activity to do, and an important aim to attain. Giving the dog a routine is highly essential than you may think. Dogs had been initially breeded by human beings to do basic activities, such as herding sheep, guarding assets and shielding human beings. Many puppies/dog today haven't had any primary activity to do, and this often resulted in boredom and neurotic behavior.

Primary obedience education, and ongoing training sessions, offers the dog an essential activity to do. This is particularly vital for high power breeds like german shepherds and border collies. Training periods are an outstanding way for these high eccentric dogs or puppies to burn up their extra power and genuinely enjoy themselves.

The art of incorporating playtime into your dog schooling or training sessions is a fantastic way to prevent both yourself and your dog from being bored. Continually have it in mind to play with your dog as it helps to facilitate and reinforce the all-crucial bond between you as the percent chief and your dog.

CHAPTER 4

Puppy/Dog Head Collar Training

The head collar has become an increasingly more popular dog training system within a couple of years. The mild chief and the halti are the most famous manufacturers of head collar in the market, however there are many different manufacturers of the simple head collar idea.

Many people find the mild chief less difficult to master than the halti, and further the mild chief is designed to lock across the dog's neck. The style of this design is that supposing the dog is in some way capable of wriggling out of the muzzle, it is still wearing a collar. This safety function is very important, especially at some stage in training outside or in lesson conditions. On the other hand, the halti gives higher control of the dog, and because of this it's far often preferred whilst running with very aggressive puppies.

Training a dog with a head collar has a number of benefits over training with a traditional or schooling collar. For one aspect, head collars are frequently easier to use for starting dog trainers than education collars. Head collars are also pretty powerful at stopping dogs from pulling, or controlling and restraining puppies that have a tendency to pull.

Head collars can also be quite powerful at

controlling dogs in tough situations, which includes controlling a dog that wants to be with different dogs. Most owners realize a few situations in which their puppies are hard to control, and head collars may be quite effective at controlling these unstable conditions.

Head collars can be excellent for controlling dogs that are very sturdy, or for running with a dog in a place that includes exceptional distractions. For example, head collars are first-rate for when your dog is on an outing, or in an area where there could be different dogs and different distractions.

Even though a head collar can be a high-quality device, it must not be used as a substitute for powerful dog education. A head collar is simplest when it's most utilized in line with sturdy and realistic dog training methods, including reward schooling and other styles of fantastic reinforcement.

Dangers of head collars

Despite the fact that head collars have many advantages, they've a few dangers as well. For one factor, head collars generally tend to make many dogs dependent on the system, and then they quickly examine the difference among their everyday collar and the head collar, and regulate their conduct therefore.

In addition, a few dogs, in particular those not accustomed to wearing a head collar, dislike sporting it and paw at it, try to rub it off or pull excessively. If your dog exhibits this behavior, the pleasant way is to maintain it is to continue till it learns to simply accept the collar. An awesome alternative is to have the dog sit down by way of pulling down at the dog's head.

Any other disadvantage of the top collar is the reaction of many human beings towards it. Many humans assume that a head collar is a muzzle, and react to the dog as if it can chunk. While this is not always a disorder of the head collar, many humans do find it tough.

Dog education with a head collar is much like schooling with a schooling collar or some other device. Whilst the head collar may be a crucial and useful tool, it's very crucial to use it appropriately, comply with all package deal commands, and to combine its use with strong education strategies. The eventual goal of dog education with a head collar is to have the dog behave well with the everyday collar as it does with the specialized head collar.

CHAPTER 5

Training Collar or Choke collar

The primary dog training collar is known by many names, which include choke collar, choke chain, training collar, correction collar and slip collar. These training collars are a number of the popular and most typically used gear with each newbie and expert dog running shoes.

While a training collar is an effective device, like any device it must be used nicely if you want it to be effective for you and secure for the dog. A few of the most essential issues when using the training collar are:

- **How the collar suits the dog;** It is essential that the training collar be nicely suited for the dog. A properly geared up training collar is less complicated to use and safer for the dog.

- **Putting the training collar on nicely:** there is a right and an incorrect way to a healthy training collar and if wrongly used, will make it ineffective and probably risky.

- **The proper use of collar:** A training collar ought to be used as a sharp reminder for the dog, not as punishment. It's far crucial that constant pressure be avoided with the use of a training collar.

- **The burden of the chain and the dimensions of the links on the training collar:** It is crucial that the load of the chain be suitable to the size and weight of the dog.

- **The location of the collar on the dog:** It's very essential to properly place the collar on the dog.

The Importance of a well fitted Training Collar

Figuring out if the training collar is the right size is distinctly easy. The precise size of the training collar has to match securely, yet without difficulty over the dog's head. It's very crucial that the training collar should not fit too tightly, however it should not be too free also. A training collar that is too tight can be too difficult to position on. On the other hand, a training collar that is too free can accidentally fall off the dog's head when it lowers its head.

It's also important to understand that a training collar that is too lengthy for the dog requires an amazing deal of finesse to apply nicely. A collar that is too long can nevertheless be used, however it's going to require more ability on the part of the handler.

Proper sizing and measurement of the dog for a training collar

It's very exceptional to measure the dog's neck with a tape line, and then add 2 to 3 inches to the dimension. So if your dog has a neck 12" in diameter, you will need to buy a training collar that is 14" in length. Chain slip collars are usually sized in two inch increments.

While fitting a training collar, the part of the chain that is connected to the leash needs to be on the head of the dog's neck. With this type of arrangement, the collar releases instantly as the leash is loosened. Training collars by design have a way of making the collar tight and free in a quick manner. Tightening the collar is the first part of the correction, and making it unfastened is the second part of the correction.

If the part of the training collar that is connected to the leash is not at the top of the dog's neck, the collar can nevertheless be made tight, however it will not return back to a loose state effortlessly.

The consistent pressure on the dog's neck initiates a counter reaction on the part of the animal, and the dog will quickly learn to pull and stress towards the leash.

In the end, it's far vital to buy a training collar that is properly made and robust. Buying an excessive excellent training collar, slip collar or choke collar is essential to the safety of yourself and your dog.

If the worst happens, and your dog's training collar does spoil, it's very crucial to not panic. Most puppies might be unaware that they have damaged the collar, at the least for a few minutes. In most cases, in case you act as if the leash remains connected, you could probably get control of your dog again swiftly.

When securing a loose dog, the best strategy is to make a short slip leash by using the snap on the leash and slipping it over the dog's head. It isn't always an excellent approach, but it's going to work.

CHAPTER 6

Dog Leash & Collar Training

There are many specific kinds of dog training, and finding the one that works exceptionally for you is crucial for growing a dog that is a gifted, loyal and devoted member of the family.

All strategies of dog training points to reinforcing the relationship among dog and handler, and the success of a training program is getting the respect of the dog. Fortuitously, dogs are restless by nature so they are looking out for leaders to help them manage the anxiety, and to comply with the direction of those leaders.

Each leash/collar and reward training has been around for a very long time, and have its effectiveness tested over the years. The sort of training that works nice varies from dog to dog and from breed to breed. It's far vital to keep in mind that every breed of dog has its own specific features, bolstered via loads of years of selective breeding.

Just like human being; the personalities of dogs varies, even within same breeds. You, as the owner of the dog should recognize better than everyone else which style of dog education will work well for your dog, so it's far vital to work with the teacher you choose to achieve your aim of a motivated, obedient and pleasant dog.

Leash and collar education is an excellent way to accomplish many kinds of dog training, specifically in conditions wherein the dog must have a high level of reliability. For instance, puppies that have crucial activities to do, which includes rescue dogs, police dogs and protection dogs, commonly benefit from leash and collar education.

In leash and collar education, various levels of pressure may be used, ranging from moderate activities with the leash to the very harsh corrections. The measure of correction used must be appropriate to the scenario, considering when the use of an excessive amount of correction, or too little, could be useful or unnecessary.

In a collar and leash based totally dog training application, firstly the dog is taught a selected conduct, typically with the leash. After the dog has been verified that it knows the command, the leash is then used to correct the dog if it disobeys, or while it makes a mistake. *The leash is the principle shape of controlling and communicating with the dog in leash and collar training.*

During the use of leash and collar training, the dog should be trained to believe the handler and take delivery of his or her directions without question. In order for the dog to be completely educated, the handler ought to show the consequences to the dog when it assumes a posture or function she or he does not want it to take. This does not imply the use of pressure; however it does usually require some level of bodily manipulation. This manipulation is most effortlessly and safely accomplished using the principle tool of leash and collar education.

It's far vital for each dog instructor to remember the fact that the leash is absolutely a device. At the same time as the leash is a critical device in this form of education, it is critical for the dog instructor to devise a good way to finally gain the right outcome with the use of some similar equipment available at hand.

Even when the simplest gear at hand is the owner's

body and talent, the dog should be willing to obey. Developing a pacesetter/follower courting among handler and dog is still very vital, and it is important to apply the leash as a device and not a crutch. A properly skilled dog ought to be willing to obey whether or not the leash is present or not.

How to Educate Your Dog with a Training Collar & Leash

The leash and training collar is the most fundamental piece of device utilized in training a dog. The use of the leash and collar properly is important to successful dog training. The training collar is designed to hold a selected amount of strain every time the leash is tightened. The quantity of pressure placed on the leash controls the amount of strain placed on the training collar, and the stress may be adjusted according to how the dog responds.

How every dog responds to training with the leash and training collar is quite variable. A few puppies barely react the first time they come across a collar and leash, even as others fight this extraordinary contraption with all their might. It's far crucial to recognize how your very own dog reacts, and to evolve your education application as needed.

The first part of training with collar and leash is direction. Getting a high-quality properly-made schooling collar that will direct your dog nicely. There are many kinds of training collars and leashes in the market. The most critical thing is to pick one that is strong and nicely made. The ultimate thing you need to do is chase your dog down after it has damaged its collar.

The length of the collar has to be inches longer than the circumference of the dog's neck. It's highly crucial to correctly measure the dog's neck with the use of a measuring tape. With a view to get a correct size, you should make sure that the tape isn't tight around the dog's neck.

Maximum training collars come in even sizes, so that you must measure up to the subsequent size in case your dog's neck is of a typical variety. It is important that the chain that is attached to the collar be placed on the top of the dog's neck. This is where the training collar is designed to assimilate great stress.

The capacity to apply various degrees of strain and to relieve that strain immediately is what makes the training collar such a powerful device. It commonly takes new customers a while to get used to using the training collar, and a few styles of training collar require greater finesse than others. In case you are unsure which collar to opt for, make sure to ask an expert dog trainer, or the management personnel at your neighborhood pet store for help.

After you've become acquainted with the way the training collar works, it's time to begin the use of it to teach your dog to stroll nicely on a lead. The properly trained dog is one that will walk at his owner's side on a loose lead, neither lagging behind nor charging in advance.

The properly trained dog will also vary its tempo to satisfy that of its handler. Under no circumstances does the handler have to be compelled to change his or her pace to fit that of the dog.

If the dog does begin to walk ahead, it is vital to correct the dog right away by giving a quick tug at the leash. This could give the dog an excellent reminder that it needs to change its tempo. It's crucial to quickly relieve the strain as soon as the dog responds. The training collar is designed to relieve stress as soon as the leash is loosened.

Most dog will immediately respond to corrections via an awesome, properly used training collar. If the dog no longer responds as directed, it is crucial to use more pressure. This will be particularly useful for big dogs or the ones who've pre-existing conduct or manipulative problems. In case you are nevertheless unable to get a response out of your dog, it is possible you are using a training collar that isn't big enough for your dog. If you think this could be the case, be sure to seek an expert recommendation earlier.

How to Coach a Dog to simply accept its Collar & Leash

Getting your dog to know how to walk on a collar and leash is the basis of this education for each domestic dog. Till the dog has found how to accept the collar and leash, it will not be possible to perform any extra training.

The first step towards getting the dog to accept the collar and leash is to find a collar that suits the dog nicely. It's very crucial that the collar be neither too light nor too heavy, neither too skinny nor too thick. A collar that is too mild for the dog may be easily damaged, while a collar that is too heavy can be uncomfortable for the dog to put on. It's also crucial that the width of the shade be suitable for the scale of the dog.

Determining the proper length of the collar is pretty cool. Definitely wrap a tape or a string lightly across the dog's neck to get an accurate size. It is vital that the tape measure not be tight, simply roomy.

Most collars are sized two inch increments, so that you may additionally need to measure as much as get a well sized collar. For example, if the dog has a 13" neck, you will buy a 14" collar, and so on.

After you've purchased the suitable collar, the following step is to put it on the dog and allow it to wear it around the house.

Do not be dismayed if the dog whines, paws at the collar or in any other case attempts to cast it off. That is ordinary; the dog doesn't have to be punished for it. It's far satisfactory to simply ignore the dog and permit it to exercise its own expressions with the collar.

The dog ought to be allowed to wear the collar 24 hours to get used to the feel of the collar on its neck. After the dog has accepted the collar nicely, it's time to start introducing the leash. A lightweight leash works nice for this process.

Likewise attach the leash to the dog's collar and allow it to walk around the house with it. The dog must be supervised for the duration of this procedure if you want to make certain it doesn't get the leash caught on anything. Getting the leash stuck or snagged may want to frighten the dog and create a leash phobia that will be tough to conquer.

At the beginning, the leash needs to simply be connected for a couple of minutes at a time. It is critical to connect the leash at happy times, which include playtime, meal time, and so on.

It's very vital for the dog to associate the leash with glad things. When the leash isn't always attached to the dog, it is a superb idea to keep it close to the dog's meals and water bowls. The dog needs to be encouraged to understand the leash, and to discover that it isn't always something to fear.

After the dog is used to walking round with the leash attached. Allow the dog to stroll around. If the dog bumps into the leash, simply permit it to react and flow as it goes. *The aim of this exercise is to truly permit the dog to get used to the texture of the collar and the leash.*

It's always crucial to permit the dog lots of time to get used to wearing the collar and leash before ever attempting to lead it. It is fine to carry out this exercise in the house or different surroundings where the dog feels safe and secure. After the dog is at ease and content on foot on the leash in the house, it is okay to take it outdoors. It's far best to make those out of doors journeys very short at the start, and to extend them slowly over time. Some dogs take to the collar and leash without delay, while others may require additional time.

Training your Dog to Get Used to Collar & Leash

Walking on a collar and leash is an essential skill that each dog ought to understand. Even the first-class trained dog must by no means be taken outside the house or yard without a strong collar and leash. Even if your dog is skilled flawlessly to go off leash, accidents and distractions do take place, and a collar, with proper identification attached, is the exceptional way to be sure you will get your loved one again.

Of course before you can educate your new dog to simply accept a leash; it should first learn how to spot a collar. The first step is to pick a collar that fits the dog nicely. It's very critical to measure the puppy's neck, and to pick out a collar size therefore. After the collar has been put on the dog, allow it to get used to it. It isn't unusual for a dog to try to tug on the collar, whine and roll or squirm when first introduced to a collar.

The best strategy is to definitely ignore the dog and let it get used to the collar. It is a mistake to both punish the dog for gambling with the collar or to encourage the behavior. Distracting the dog often helps, and playing with a favorite toy, or ingesting some favorite treats, can help the dog quickly forget that it is wearing this strange piece of gadget.

After the dog has learned to simply accept the collar, attempt including the leash. Hook the leash to the collar and genuinely sit and watch the dog. Obviously, this ought to most effectively be achieved either inside the house or in restricted outdoor vicinity. The dog should be allowed to pull the leash around on its own, but of course the owner have to maintain a near eye at the dog to make certain that the leash does not come to be snagged or hung up on something.

At first, the leash should simply be left on for a few

minutes at a time. It is a good concept to connect the leash at mealtimes, playtime and different high-quality times. That manner the dog will begin to associate the leash with good matters and look forward to it. If the dog exhibits an excessive amount of uneasiness regarding the leash, it is advisable to limit it subsequently to meals times for a while to allow it get used to it slowly. In the end, it's going to come to remember that the leash is not anything to be afraid of.

After the dog is comfortable with strolling around the residence wearing the leash, it's time for you to pick up the leash for a few minutes. You need to try and stroll with the dog on the leash; definitely maintain control of the leash and comply with the dog as it walks round. You need to try and avoid conditions where the leash turns rigid and any pulling or straining on the leash should be avoided. It's problematic for the dog to stay down. Try some video games with the collar and leash. For example, stand up and inspire your dog to stroll in your direction. Don't drag your puppy forward; inspire it to come to you. If it does, praise it profusely and praise it with a meal treat or toy. You must always attempt to make all the time spent on the leash as excellent as possible.

It is crucial to offer the dog plenty of exercise in being used to the leash inside the house. It's very nice to do plenty of work inside the home, considering that it's secure surroundings with few distractions. After the puppy is comfortable on foot inside and on a leash, it's time to start going outside, starting of in small enclosed vicinity like a fenced Yard. After the puppy has mastered walking flippantly outside on a leash, it is time to visit a few places where there are extra distractions. You could need first of all a place like a neighbor's yard. Walking your new dog across the community is a good way to introduce your pals to the new puppy, even as giving the puppy some good petting in fending off distractions and focusing on his leash training.

Dogs ever so often exhibit bad conduct with their leashes, such as biting or chewing at the leash. To discourage this kind of conduct, try applying a bit of sour apple, tabasco sauce or similar substance (simply make certain the substance you apply is not toxic to puppies). This approach commonly convinces dogs that chewing the leash is a bad idea.

Teaching your Dog to not pull at the leash

Pulling on the leash is one of the most common misbehaviors seen on all varieties of dogs. Dogs and pet dogs alike can regularly be seen taking their owners for walks, in preference to the opposite custom. Pulling at the leash may be quite more than a stressful dependancy. Leash pulling can lead to getting out of hand situation in the case of a wreck in the collar or leash, and an out of control, off leash dog may be both unfavourable and perilous to itself and to others.

Leash pulling can result from a diffusion of various

things. In some cases, the dog may additionally be so excited to head for a walk that it is unable to control itself. In most cases, the dog sees itself as the leader and it truely takes the *"leadership position"* at the front of the dog handler.

If excitement is the incentive for leash pulling, in reality giving the dog a few minutes to relax can frequently be of massive help. Stand with the dog on the leash for a pair of minutes and let the initial pleasure of the upcoming stroll skip. After the initial pleasure has worn off, many puppies are willing to stroll calmly on their leash.

If the problem is out of control, however, a little

restraint can be useful. All dog education starts off evolved with the owner setting up him or herself as the alpha dog, or leader, without this simple respect and information, no powerful training can occur. For dogs displaying these kinds of control issues, a step back to fundamental obedience command is necessary. Those dogs can frequently be helped via a formal obedience faculty structure. The dog trainer will of course be sure to educate the handler as well as the dog, and any thorough dog trainer will insist on working with the dog owner as well as the dog.

The idea of coaching the dog to walk calmly on the leash is coaching it to evenly be given the collar and lead. A dog that is bouncing up and down even as the collar is being put on will not stroll well. Start by instructing your dog to sit, and insist that it takes a seat nonetheless while the collar is placed on. If the dog starts to rise, or takes off on its own after the collar is on, be sure to sit it back and backtrack it at once. Best start the walk after the dog has sat and has the collar placed on and continues to take a seat evenly because the leash is attached.

Once the leash is connected, it's very vital to make the dog stroll calmly towards the door. If the dog jumps or surges beforehand, gently correct it with a tug of the leash and get it back to a sitting position. Make the dog stay and then continue again. Repeat this system till the dog is on foot calmly by your side.

Repeat the above method until you reach the door. The dog should not be allowed to surge out of the door, or to tug you by the open door. If the dog begins this conduct, take back the dog into the house and make it sit quietly until it can be trusted to walk through the door nicely. Beginning the walk while in control is important to developing a properly-mannered dog.

As you begin your stroll, it's very crucial to keep the attention of the dog centered on you at all times. Do not forget, the dog have to look to you for direction, not take the lead itself. When taking walks, it's very crucial to forestall often. Every time you forestall, your dog must stop. Getting into the habit of asking your dog to sit down each time is a great way to keep your dog's interest focused on you. Make certain your dog is looking at you, and then go off again. If the dog begins to surge beforehand, at once forestall and ask the dog to sit. Repeat this technique until the dog is consistently staying at your side. Whenever the dog does what you ask it to, ensure you give it a treat, a toy or simply a reward.

Keep in mind that if your dog pulls on the leash and also you ensure to stop the stroll because you're inadvertently correcting that undesirable behavior. Puppies learn whether or not you're coaching them, and gaining knowledge of the wrong things now will make it difficult knowing the right one. It's far essential to be consistent on your expectancies. Whenever the dog starts to drag ahead of time, without delay stop and make the dog sit down. Remember to have the dog take a seat quietly until its focus is purely on you. Then start out again, ensuring at once to forestall strolling if the dog surges ahead.

Puppy/Dog off-leash Training

Many dog owners worry about giving their 4 legged companions the freedom of going off leash, but it's very important not to hurry that essential step. Puppies ought to be allowed off their leash after they have come to be masters of all of the simple obedience instructions, such as taking walks at your heel, sitting and remaining under command.

Any other ability that needs to be completely mastered before the dog can be taken off the leash is the *'come'* command. Even supposing the dog can heel, sit and live perfectly, if it can not be relied upon to return while called, it isn't prepared up to be taken off the leash.

Taking any dog off the leash, in particular in a hectic, crowded region, or one with a variety of site visitors, is a large step and not one to be taken lightly. It's far crucial to accurately test your dog in safe surroundings before taking it off the leash. After all, the leash is the primary tool of control. You have to be very positive and depend on your voice commands for control before removing the leash.

After the dog has been educated to recognize the take a seat and stay command, and responds to instructions, it's very crucial to challenge the dog with numerous distractions. It is a good idea to start by introducing other people, different animals, or both, while the dog is in a secure surrounding like a fenced backyard. Have a chum or neighbor stand simply outside the fence while you hold your dog at the leash. Because the friend or family member walks around outside the fence, watch your dog's reactions closely. If it starts off, pull on the leash fast and tug until it returns.

Repeat this exercise until the dog will reliably remain at your side. After this, you may try losing the leash, and ultimately getting rid of the leash and repeating the distraction. It is crucial to vary the distractions, which include introducing different animals, different humans, traffic, rolling balls, etc.

After your dog is capable of staying still in the face of distractions, begin introducing the *'come command'* with distractions in the vicinity. Attempt to invite some of the neighbors, and their dogs over to play with each other. Because the puppies are playing in the fenced yard, try calling your dog. While the dog comes to you, make sure you praise it a lot, and perhaps a meal reward. After the dog has been rewarded, straight away allow him to go playing again. Repeat this several times in the course of the day, ensuring on every occasion to praise the dog and at once allow him to move back to its species.

After the dog has apparently mastered coming when called on its own, strive locating a nearby dog park or similar region where you could practice along with your dog. It's far important to make the location small, or to pick a fenced location incase you lose control of the dog. In case you cannot find a fenced location, pick an area well away from people and cars. Exercise together with your dog by allowing it to play with other dogs, or simply sniffing around, then calling your dog. When it comes to you, without delay praise it, then allow it resume its preceding activities. Doing this may teach the dog that coming to you is the best alternative and the one most probably to bring both rewards and praise at all times.

After the dog has constantly mastred the capacity to come when called upon, even when there are numerous distractions around, it is safe to allow it time without work leash. Off leash time must by no means be an unsupervised time. It's far crucial that you are aware of what your dog is doing at all times. It is simple for a dog to get into trouble fast, so you ought to always keep a fixed eye on it, whether it's chasing squirrels in the park, playing with different dogs, or just chasing a ball with the neighbor's kids.

CHAPTER 7

Dog Obedience Lessons

Obedience training is one of the most essential training and probabaly the only thing any owner can do for his or her dog. An obedient and trained dog is a satisfied, productive and secure member of the family, at the same time an untrained dog can be harmful and even dangerous.

Dog are designed by way nature to follow leaders, and to look for that leadership in you. As most animals, dog certainly observe the instructions of their handler. In the absence of the handler, the dog may exhibit this function itself. Dogs that see themselves as leaders because the handler is human can emerge as uncooperative, unfavourable and even dangerous.

Precisely, obedience training opens up crucial strains of conversation among handler and dog. The idea of any obedience training program is to gain the cooperation and respect of the animal. This respect cannot be exerted via difficult handling strategies or mistreatment. It needs to be a substitute and must be earned via management and proper education strategies.

Fundamental obedience training includes coaching the dog what to do and what not to do. With regards to preferred behaviors, it's far crucial for the dog to understand and reply to primary commands, including heeling while on foot, stopping on command, sitting while directed, coming while called and staying in whens the handler directs.

The list of what not to do is likewise vital in terms of obedience training. Some of the don'ts of obedience training encompass; *not jumping on human beings, not charging in advance while taking walks and, not chewing the furnishings or your property, and not getting out of control while exposed to lesson situations.*

In essence, obedience training entails establishing the social hierarchy that is as critical to puppy as adult dogs. While your dog follows your obedience instructions such as; *come, stay, take a seat, heel, etc.,* it is displaying compliance and submissiveness. This is the same type of behavior a submissive member of a wild dog pack might display to the alpha dog in that group.

As with every sort of dog training, it is crucial that obedience training sessions be amusing and rewarding for both dog and handler. A glad, healthy dog can be fun to manage, and maintaining the excitement throughout the training sessions will make life easier for both you and your dog. Obedience training has many benefits for the dog in addition to the handler. For one component, a nicely-skilled, obedient dog can be given a greater amount of freedom than an untrained dog. For instance, a dog that has been nicely trained to respond positively when called can correctly enjoy a few off leash play time at the neighborhood park.

There is continually a debate over whether it is less difficult to teach obedience to puppy or older dogs. The fact is that both dogs and puppy may be efficaciously trained to be willing, obedient companions. It is easier to educate puppies and young dog than it is to retrain dog that have developed conduct issues. Even troublesome dogs can be efficaciously retrained on the practice of basic obedience training and control concepts.

When training dog on obedience, it's far important to remember that puppy generally have a shorter attention span than full grown dogs. It is crucial, therefore to begin training classes quickly from the start. It is also crucial to have plenty of playtimes with different dog, puppies and different animals, as well as lots of various humans. Proper socialization is very crucial to creating a safe, healthful and satisfied dog.

There are many obedience training institutions held in all parts of the country, and new dog and dog owners are encouraged to join one of these institutions. No longer does a simple dog kindergarten and dog obedience class offer crucial structure for the dog, but it gives room for correct socialization of the dog as well.

The importance of rewards

Rewards simply can be the most crucial motivator in dog training. Obedience training using rewards and other fantastic reinforcements has long been identified as the easiest technique of achieving success in most dog and getting the best possible results.

Making obedience training entertaining, and even making it a bit of a game, may be very essential to sustaining both the dog and the handler's interest and willingness to learn. Incorporating a period of playtime at the beginning and end of each training class will ensure that every session starts off strong and ends in an excellent note.

The most simple of all obedience instructions is heeling, or taking walks with the handler on a free leash. That is typically the first obedience conduct that is taught, and it's also an easy one to teach through reward training. Start by fitting the dog with a quality, well geared up training leash and collar. If you are uncertain of how to fit the training collar, make certain to invite a dog instructor or the supervisor at the shop where the device was purchased.

Start on foot with the dog, constantly being aware of the dog's function relative to your training. If the dog starts to charge beforehand, gently pull on the leash. This will deliver a gentle reminder for the dog to slow down. It could be vital to use extra pressure at the beginning till the dog learns to simply accept the correction.

If the dog starts off by falling behind, lightly urge the dog ahead, using a lure, or a favorite toy. It would be very beneficial when coaching the dog to walk at your pace. To keep it at the preferred position, it has to study the preferred place and quickly too.

Constantly make certain to offer lots of reward, treats, toys and different rewards whilst the dog does what is expected of him. Dog understand best with the aid of superb reinforcement.

Effective reinforcement means that when the animal does what the handler wants, it gets a reward, which may be something from a pat on the head to a treat with a favorite toy. At the start of the training, even the slightest act to please the owner ought to be rewarded.

Training with use of reprimands and punishment isn't always nearly as powerful as training by means of rewards. Dogs can become discouraged and harassed by excessive amounts of punishment and reprimands. Reprimands may be required from time to time, to dangerous behaviors like chasing or biting, for example, however reprimands have to be brief and without delay applied to the trouble at hand. After the immediate danger has passed, the training must continue with reward based education and positive reinforcement.

For instance, if you catch your dog chewing the furniture or other object, without delay offer the dog a straight "no" or "stop" and take the item away. Then without delay provide the dog one of its toys or other items that it is allowed to chunk on, and reward the dog enthusiastically while it is taking the toy. This may train the dog to associate chewing a few objects, like his toys, with reward, and chewing irrelevant items with reprimand.

It is very essential for the dog to make those relations, considering the fact that it is very tough to trade terrible habits after they are formed. It's a lot simpler to teach right obedience behaviors at the beginning than it is to retrain a difficult dog afterward. This doesn't suggest that retraining is impossible; it truly means that it's extra tough. Coaching a puppy, or an older dog, to grasp the behaviors you value, which includes coming when called to, sitting on command, strolling at your pace, chewing on toys, and so on, is the idea of a successful dog training.

CHAPTER 8

Lucky Dog Reward Lessons

Reward training is regularly seen as the most cutting-edge technique of training a dog, however reward lesson is probably a whole lot older than other techniques of dog training. It is possible that reward training for dogs has been around so long as there have been dogs to teach. Early people probably used a few casual kind of reward training when taming the wolf domestic dogs that subsequently evolved into modern-day dogs.

What's called reward schooling or training for dogs nowadays has enjoyed top notch recognition for 10 to 15 years.

Many prized training fanatics are less captivated

with different methods of dog training, which include the conventional leash and collar method. However, the satisfactory method for training any dog is often a mixture of leash/collar education and reward training.

Furthermore, a training approach that works flawlessly for one dog can work differently for another, and vice versa. A few dog respond fabulously to reward training and in no way to leash and collar training, at the same time some others may respond to leash/collar education and not feel encouraged by means of reward education. Most dog fall someplace inside the middle of these extremities.

Clicker training is one of the maximum popular

sorts of reward education in recent times. At the same time as clicker schooling is not the answer for every dog; it may be a remarkably powerful approach of training many dog. In clicker training, the dog is taught to associate a clicking sound with reward, like a treat. The instructor clicks the clicker when the dog does something good, accompanied immediately with a treat. Ultimately, the dog learns to reply to the clicker on its own.

Most reward training makes use of a few types of meal reward, or a reward that is associated with getting food. In most cases, complex behaviors can easily adopt the use of this type of high quality reinforcement, and you'll find that the individuals who train dogs for movies and television use reward training almost solely.

Reward training is used in all sorts of dog training, along with police and army trainings. Maximum fragrance detection, monitoring and police dog are trained on the use of a few form of reward training. Reward training is also a very powerful method to educate various basic obedience instructions.

Reward training often involves enticing the dog into the position preferred by the instructor. The lure is used to get the dog to carry out the desired conduct on its own free will.

It makes an excellent deal of sense to get the dog to perform the preferred conduct without any physical intervention on the part of the handler. Getting the dog to perform a conduct without physical contact is vital.

After the dog has achieved the desired conduct, it is given a reward, also known as a fine reinforcement. Treats are often used as reinforcers, but reward, such as "good dog" or a pat on the head, can also be an effective reward.

Having a dog that has been reward trained to be a reliable dog is crucial, especially while the dog has a crucial program, like police patrol or drug detection, to do. Because of this it's far essential to get the dog accustomed to running around in the face of distractions, and to properly socialize the animal to both humans and different animals.

Many dog owners make the mistake of only

training the dog within the house or lower backyard, and only while the handler is there. This allows you to end up a reliably skilled accomplice; the dog must be taken outdoors, out of the confines of its protection region and introduced to lesson conditions.

It's also crucial to train the dog to take note of the handler always. By keeping your eyes away from the dog means having control of the dog. Reward training could be very powerful at getting the honour and the attention of the dog when used nicely.

Treats and Food Primarily based Rewards

Training with treats and other food primarily based rewards is a first rate way to encourage your dog and speed the training method simultaneously. Most dog are quite motivated by using meal rewards, and most animal schools use this kind of fine reinforcement to train all varieties of animals, together with tigers, lions, and elephants and even residence cats.

It's advisable to start a treat based total training consultation, but it is a good concept to check the dog to ensure that food will motivate him via the consultation. Begin with the dog's everyday supper time by taking a bit of its meals and waving it in the front of the dog's nose. If the dog shows an enthusiasm for the meal, then it's best to start the training. If the dog indicates little interest or none in any respect, it is advisable to do away with the education till some other time. Don't be afraid to put off dinner time for you to pique the dog's hobby in training. The benefits of proper education will outweigh any delay in feeding.

It's very normal to get the dog used to normal feedings, as opposed to leaving food out all the time. Not only does loose feeding encourage the dog to overeat and boom the chances of weight problems, but a free fed dog may in no way be fully prompted in reward primarily based education.

The *'Come when Called'* Training

Once your dog has shown interest for the meals presented to it, it's time to begin this education/training. Since you already gave your dogs undivided attention through showing it food, now is a top notch time to start. Deliver the dog some portions of food right away, after which go up again a few steps. While holding the meals with your hand, beckon it with the *"come right here"* command. While the dog comes to you, reward him lavishly and provide him a few portions of meals.

After the dog is coming to you effortlessly, add *"take a seat"* command and maintain the collar before you supply the meals. After the *take a seat* command is mastered, other commands, and even a few hints, may be added. Meals based reinforcement education is the pleasant way to educate a selection of essential behaviors.

One true exercising command is the *take a seat* command. This exercise can start with the owner keeping a foot on the dog, then preventing and asking the dog to sit. After the dog is sitting quietly, the owner backs away and asks the dog to stay. Preferably the dog should continue to stay until called by the owner, despite the fact that the leash is dropped. At the end of the exercise, the owner calls the dog. While the dog goes to the owner, it gets food and reward from the owner. This exercise should be repeated numerous times, until the dog is reliably coming when called.

It's far essential to keep the training sessions quick, especially in the beginning, to hold the dog from becoming bored, and from ingesting its whole meal in the form of treats. After the dog has been responding frequently, the treats and food rewards can be slowly reduced. It's far essential to still offer these food rewards, but don't offer much. After some time, it's not vital to present the dog treats each single time he responds as requested. In essence, it needs to only be essential for the dog to get hold of a food treat one out of 5 instances it comes when commanded. The alternative four successes can be rewarded with praise and scratches.

As soon as the dog is aware of the basics of the *"come right here"* command, the simple command may be improved, and many video games can be created. These varieties of video games may be remarkable fun for owner and dog alike, in addition to a tremendous get to know experience. A few off leash work can be added as well, however it's far more excellent to begin with the dog in a safe surrounding, along with a fenced lower back yard. For variety, you can attempt taking the dog to other secure environments, inclusive of a pal's residence, a neighbor's fenced backyard or a neighborhood dog park. Try leaving the dog free in those safe places, and exercise the come command. Usually praise the dog significantly, scratch it at the back of the ears and tell it what an awesome dog it is. The purpose must be to make coming to the owner a big deal.

The Use of Reward Training

Training dog with the use of high-quality reinforcement and reward training has long been diagnosed as both enormously effective for the owner and a superb experience for the dog. Effective reinforcement education is so essential that it's far the easiest approach used to teach dangerous animals like lions and tigers to work in circuses and within the film and TV enterprise. Proponents of nice reinforcement vouch on the effectiveness of their techniques, and it's far authentic that a good sized majority of dog respond nicely to these training techniques.

One reason why high quality reinforcement training is so powerful is that it makes use of rewards to teach the dog what is expected of it. When the dog performs the desired conduct, it is provided with a reward, most usually within the form of a food treat however it can be a scratch behind the ears, a rub underneath the chin or a pat on the head as well. The crucial aspect is that the dog is rewarded always for doing the right thing.

Reward education has become increasingly popular in recent years, however there are a few sort of reward education among human beings and dog that has been going on for a long time if not hundreds of years.

In understanding what makes reward training so effective, some knowledge of the history of humans and dog could be very helpful. The earliest dog have been likely wolf dog that had been tamed and used by early humans for safety from predators, as alarm structures and later for guarding and herding cattle. It's far viable that the wolf pups that made the best companions had been the most without apparent training, or it's very possible that those early dog were orphaned or deserted wolf pups. Noting their starting place, there's little doubt today that the huge sort of dogs we see these days have their starting place in the wolf.

Wolf packs, like packs of untamed dogs, perform on a strict P.C. Hierarchy. Due to the fact that wolf and dog packs hunt as a set, this type of hierarchy, and the cooperation it brings, is vital to the survival of the species. Every dog is aware of its place in the P.C., and in the event of death or injury, the hierarchy, as soon as set up, hardly ever adjusts.

Each dog, consequently, is highly wired with the aid of nature to look to the P.C. leader for steerage. The basis of every proper dog education, which includes reward based education, is for the handler to set him or herself up as the absolute leader. The chief handler is greater than simply the dominant dog, or the only who tells all of the subordinates what to do. More importantly, the chief gives management and safety, and his or her leadership is essential to the achievement and survival of the pack. It's far essential for the dog to see itself as part of a P.C., to recognize the human as the chief of that pack, and to respect his or her authority. Some dogs are a good deal less complicated to dominate than others. In case you watch a set of dogs playing for a while, you'll quickly recognize the dominant and submissive personalities.

A dog with a more submissive personality will typically be less complicated to train with the use of fantastic reinforcement, on the grounds that it won't want to challenge the handler for leadership. Even dominant dogs respond thoroughly to high quality reinforcement. There are, in fact few dog that don't reply well to high quality reinforcement, additionally known as reward training. Fantastic reinforcement is also a nice way to retrain a dog that has conduct problems, especially one which has been abused. Getting the trust and loyalty of an abused dog may be very hard, and superb reinforcement is higher than another training technique at creating this vital bond.

Irrespective of what type of dog you're working with, there are possibilities that it can be helped with effective reinforcement training strategies. Base your training strategies on appreciation and reward rather than intimidation and worry, it is the best way to get the most from any dog.

CHAPTER 9

Dogs' Crate, Potty & House Training

House training is one of the maximum essential elements of training any dog to be a valued part of the family. As with many other aspects of dog education, the best way to house train a dog is to use the dog's very own nature to your advantage.

The splendid thing about dogs, and the element which can make house education a great deal less difficult, is that dogs are instinctively very easy animals. Dogs would as an alternative not soil the areas where they sleep and eat. Similarly, dogs are superb at grown up behavior regarding where they like to urinate and defecate. For instance, dog that are used to going off on concrete or gravel will prefer to go off right there instead of on grass or dirt. It's far viable to use those natural dog conduct when house training your dog.

Crate Training for Dog

Crate training is one of the easiest methods of house training any dog or puppy. Crate education may be very efficient, and really effective, since it makes use of the natural instinct of the dog to reap the preferred end result of a clean house and a properly-skilled dog.

The idea of crate training is that a dog evidently strives to keep away from soiling the location where it eats and sleeps. By way of placing the dog inside the crate, this intuition is stronger. The dog will come to look at the crate as its den, and it will try to keep away from soiling its den.

The key to a successful crate education for a dog, as with other varieties of dog training, is to establish a terrific and recurrent procedure. This habit will beautify the capability of the dog to do its shitty business within the proper place, and keep away from the wrong places. It's far crucial to shower the dog with reward whenever it defecates in the set up lavatory location, and not to express frustration or anger when the dog makes a mistake.

It is important to confine the dog to a small part of the house, usually a dog proofed room, when you are not at home. The room has to contain a tender bed, fresh water and some preferred toys to save the dog from becoming bored and restless.

Crate training isn't like confining the dog to a room, however. With crate training, the dog is restricted to a crate when unsupervised. The idea is that the dog will think about this crate as its home, and will no longer want to soil its home.

While crate training, it is important to remove the dog from the crate as soon as possible after returning home, and to take the dog right away to the previously mounted rest room area. When the dog does its business in the toilet, be sure to offer plenty of reward and treats. It's very important that the dog learns to associate proper rest room techniques with appropriate things like treats and toys.

It is essential to never leave the dog in its crate for long periods of time, as this could confuse the dog and pressure it to soil its napping vicinity. The crate is surely a tool, and it ought not to be abused by way of leaving the dog in it for prolonged intervals. If the dog is left inside the crate for too long it could cause a major setback on the training by weeks if not months.

The dog ought to only be limited to the crate when you are at home during the day, because at night dogs have to relieve themselves at least forty five minutes or so. Whenever the dog is taken out; it ought to be put on a leash and without delay taken outdoors. Once it's outside the residence, the dog needs to be given 3 to 5 minutes to do its enterprise. If the dog does not do so, it must be returned to the crate.

If the dog does its business at some time in the long run, it needs to be rewarded with reward, food, play, affection and a prolonged walk or duration of play interval outside the home.

All through the crate education duration, it's very essential to preserve a daily diary of the dog's toilet activities. If the dog is on an ordinary feeding agenda, the toilet schedule ought to be regular. Having a good record of when the dog wishes to get rid of waste each day might be a big help throughout the house training process. After the dog has used its established toilet place, you will be able to provide the dog free run of the house to play and celebrate with it.

Managing shortcomings during puppy/dog crate Training

It is very crucial not to punish the dog while it makes a mistake or has a twist of fate during the crate training procedure. If there was a twist of fate, absolutely ease up. Accidents throughout house training suggest that you have provided the dog with unsupervised right of entry into the house too fast. The dog ought not to be allowed unsupervised access to the house until you can agree with its bowel and bladder behavior. If errors do occur, it is satisfactory to move again to crate education. Taking a couple of steps back will assist it to pass the house education technique, at the same time as shifting too quick could set matters back.

Setting up the Training Vicinity

The first step in house training your dog is to set up your training vicinity. A small, confined area which includes a rest room, or a part of a kitchen or garage, works satisfactory as an education area. This method of education differs from crate training. *Crate education is first-rate for dog and small dogs, but many large dogs find a crate too confining.*

It's far crucial for the owner to spend as much time in the training vicinity with his or her dog as possible. It's far vital for the owner to play with the dog within the training location, and to permit the dog to eat and sleep in that vicinity. The dog needs to be provided with a special mattress within the training location, something from a store, like mattress, a big towel in a huge container. At first, the dog may additionally go off this area, however once the dog has diagnosed it as its own space, it would be reluctant to soil it.

After the dog has gotten used to snoozing within the mattress, the owner can pass it across the residence, relocating it from room to room. When you aren't together with your dog, the dog ought to be restricted to the training area.

Potty Training for Puppy/Dog

The second part of residence training is to set up the rest room/ toilet training region for the dog. It's far vital for the dog to have a right of entry to this area every time it wishes to go off. It is also crucial for the owner to accompany the dog every time till it masters the habit of going off in the bathroom area. Ensure the dog only makes use of the mounted toilet area.

A set feeding time table makes the house education method pretty less complicated for both the owner and the dog. Feeding the dog on a normal basis will also create a regular time table for the dog's toilet behavior. Once you recognize when your dog is probably likely to defecate, it will be easy to lead the dog to the mounted bathroom vicinity.

As soon as the dog has hooked up a lavatory area and is used to it on a daily basis, it's far very vital not to confine the dog without access to the toilet place for long durations of time. This is because if the dog is unable to preserve it, it may be pressured to go off the training place. This habit could make residence training very tough.

Expanding puppy/dog house training method

After the dog is constantly going off inside the toilet area and not soiling the training ground, it is time to extend that education location to the rest of the house. This method should be performed slowly, starting with one room and slowly expanding to the rest of the house. The location has to be extended only after you are sure of the dog's capability to manage its bladder and bowels.

When you first increase the education region to an unmarked room, allow the dog to devour, play and sleep in that room, however stay close and supervise. When it isn't always possible to oversee the dog, place it back to the original training vicinity. Then, after the dog has become acquainted with the room as an extension of the authentic training area, the vicinity can be extended.

If this method is simply too long to satisfy your

needs, it can be accelerated, but it is essential to proceed carefully. It's far less difficult to face the problem up front than to restrain a problematic dog for later. One way to efficiently speed up residence training is to reward and appreciate the dog every time it uses the installed rest room region. It's also important not to punish the dog for errors. Punishment will only confuse the dog and slow down the residence training technique.

CHAPTER 10

The Do's & Don'ts of Dogs' House Training

House training a dog is very crucial for the wellbeing of both the dog and the owner. The number one reason dogs are sent to animal shelters is trouble, so it is important to look at why residence training is such a crucial issue.

It is crucial to set up a right bathroom conduct while the dog is younger, due to the fact that, this habit can last a lifetime, and be very tough to break as soon as they are learned. It's very vital for the owner to train the dog well. In most instances, proper residence education can not start till the dog is six months old. Dogs younger than this commonly lack the bowel and bladder control needed for house education.

Dogs younger than six months must be limited to a small, dog proofed room when the owner cannot supervise them. The entire floor of the room must be filled with newspapers or comparable absorbent materials, and the paper changed each time it is soiled. As the dog becomes smarter, the quantity of paper used may be decreased because the dog starts developing a preferred lavatory place. A preferred bathroom space is preferable in order to form the basis of house training.

The do's of house training your dog

- Constantly provide the dog with steady, unrestricted access to the lavatory region.

- When at home take the dog to the rest room region every forty five minutes.

- When dog supervision is not optional, you ought to be sure it can't make a mistake. This indicates confining the dog to a small area that has been thoroughly dog proofed.

- Usually offer a lavatory place that doesn't resemble anything in your home. Training the dog to dispose of on concrete, blacktop, grass or dirt is a great concept. The dog must by no means be encouraged to defecate on anything that resembles the hardwood floors, tile.

- Reward your dog every time he goes to toilet area. The dog needs to learn to associate defecating within the hooked up areas with right things, like treats, toys and reward from his owner.

- Always keep a fixed agenda when feeding your dog, a constant feeding schedule equals a regular rest room schedule.

- The use of a crate can be a massive support in helping a dog develop willpower. The concept behind crate training is that the dog will no longer want to go defecate in its mattress vicinity.

- And subsequently, it's very essential to be

patient when house training a dog. House education can take as long as many months, however it's a whole lot less complicated to house train at the right time than to restrain a problematic dog.

The don'ts of house training your dog

- By no means reprimand or punish the dog for mistakes. Punishing the dog will only cause fear and confusion.

- Do not leave meals out for the dog all night. Stick to a fixed feeding agenda as a way of making the dog's toilet schedule as constant as possible.

- Do not allow the dog freedom in the house until it has been very well house skilled.

House training is not usually the easiest aspect to do, and some dog tend to be lot difficult to teach than others. It is vital to be patient, steady and loving as you teach your dog. A rushed, apprehensive or intimidated dog will not be able to study the crucial lessons of residence training. As soon as you've gained your dog's love and respect, you'll find that house training your dog is less complicated than you ever expected.

How to Deal with the Hassle of House Training your Dog

House training is one of those problems that every dog owner needs to grapple with. In most cases, residence training is the first main milestone within the relationship between owner and dog, and it can be tough and confusing for owner and dog alike.

The best house training tactics are those who use the dog's personal instincts to the owner's advantage. Those strategies consider the dog's reluctance to soil the spots wherein he eats and sleeps. This is the idea behind house training and crate training. Dog are very interesting animals, and in nature they constantly keep away from the use of their house as rest room areas.

These types of natural training techniques commonly work very well, for young dog and older dog. Certainly, older, larger dog will want a bigger area for its den, and crate training is typically best used for larger dog and smaller dog.

While house training a dog or a domestic dog, it is vital to pay close attention to the signs the dog is sending. It's also essential to be consistent in regards to feeding times, and to offer the dog freedom to the toilet place you set up on a normal foundation.

It's very crucial to never rush the technique of house education. At the same time as few dogs are evidently simpler to educate, most owners will experience minimum shortcomings during the house training procedure. While these injuries occur, it's highly crucial not to get mad and punish the dog. Shortcomings during house training usually imply that the owner is trying to progress too quickly, or that the dog has been left alone for too long. In this case, it's best to simply take a step back and start the technique again.

It's also essential for the owner to reward the dog enthusiastically while it does its private business inside the appointed vicinity. The dog has to learn how to associate doing its private business in its toilet vicinity with right things like treats, rewards and applause.

For the duration of the house training method, the

toilet region starts off very small, as small as 1/2 of a small room in the beginning, because the dog learns to control its bladder and bowels better, and the owner learns to understand the dog's rest room desires, the toilet area can be slowly improved. It's no longer necessary to make the den area too huge too quickly. The den area needs to be enhanced slowly for the house training procedure to progress smoothly.

It is vital for the dog to be well acquainted to its den. Many dog, particularly those who've in no way been given freedom outside the owner's inspection before, together with those who have spent their lives as outdoor dog, may additionally react to the den location as though it is a prison, and continuously whine, bark and try to break out the den. It is crucial that the dog discover ways to consider its den/cage as a domestic house and no longer a cage.

One problem many dog owners forget while house training a dog is that of boredom. Boredom is surely the root cause of many conduct issues in dogs, together with chewing and other unfavorable behaviors. Boredom can also be the basic motive of problems with house training.

Dogs that are bored regularly take huge quantities of water all day, and this extra water intake can lead to the desire to urinate regularly, even in its den area. Because soiling the den area is going against the dog's nature, he can quickly become harassed and anxious, thereby setting the house training program back even further.

To prevent the dog from becoming bored while you are far from home, make certain to offer him lots of different varieties of toys, in addition to a secure and cozy area to sleep. In addition, a vigorous amount of play time can assist the dog sleep even as you are away. Further, gambling with the dog in its den area will help him bond with this area and see it as a secure, at ease space.

CHAPTER 11

Advance Dog Training

Responding immediately when called is an essential ability that every dog should exhibit, both for its personal protection and for those around it. A disobedient dog that refuses to respond when called could be hit by an automobile, get into a fight with another dog or go through a series of other bad experiences. A properly trained dog that comes when called can be taken out to play in the neighborhood park, at the seaside, at the hiking path, or anywhere else the owner and dog may also desire to go.

Simply teaching the dog to come when called is distinctly smooth and simple, and involves offering reward, treats and different perks while the dog does as its owner desires. After those simple commands known as physical training games are mastered, there are a number of fun sporting events that can be introduced to the dog as a hobby.

Turning training into an amusing game is one of the satisfactory methods to inspire dogs and handler alike. It is normal for training periods to become routine and boring, and it's highly essential to keep them from degenerating into this state.

Before beginning any meal based training workout, it is crucial to make sure that the dog is well influenced and ready to respond to instruction. Start by taking a bit of its regular food and waving it in front of the dog's nose, if the dog shows high enthusiasm for the food, it is ready to start the training. If not, it's far great to wait until the dog is in a more receptive mood.

Use treats that shows best response with primarily based training games like hide and seek or smaller pieces of cheese and liver. In other words, something your dog will love. It is great to use very small portions to keep it from over-feeding throughout the training periods.

One wonderful sport for you and any other member of the family or friend to play along with your dog is back and front don't forget. This is an extremely good exercise for teaching your dog to return

Whenever it's called by different member of the

family, dogs often find ways to only respond to at least one individual, and this will be a problem when different human beings are looking at the dog. This is one reason why professional dog handlers usually insist on working with the owner. A well skilled dog ought to learn to reply to whoever is around, not simply the owner or handler.

In a secure area like a fenced yard, one individual calls the dog and asks it to sit and stay till another person asks it to come back. While the dog responds to the command to come back, it is rewarded with a treat. Most dog respond superbly to this exercise and love playing this sport. While playing the back and forth bear in mind that it is critical that only the individual that called the dog be allowed to give it a treat.

After the dog has mastered the back and forth sport, the people in the sport can start to spread out, accordingly turning it into a game of hide and seek. Every time they call the dog to return, they spread out faraway from where they began. As the game keeps up, one person could be at one end of the residence, whilst another can be at the other end. What makes the game so amusing for the dog is that it must search out the person to get the treat, in place of truly walking up to someone in plain sight. This type of game appeals to several of the dog's herbal instincts. In spite of everything, dogs are obviously hunting animals, and looking for food is second nature to them.

Keeping your Dog Motivated

Keeping the dog focused and motivated during training isn't alwys easy. Dog can be easily distracted, and it's far necessary not to allow the training periods to be disrupted by boredom. Making training fun for the dog and the human handler likewise is important to developing a happy, well-adjusted and nicely skilled dog.

Providing random nice incentives for the duration of the day is a superb way to keep the interest of the dog. Doing things the dog enjoys, like strolling in the park, driving in a car, and playing with different dog, is a notable way to keep the dog's interest and reward it for small successes.

For example, in other to reward the dog for coming to you, ask the dog to come to you without giving any clues like a stroll, a car trip, or different treats. After the dog has come to you and obediently sat down, connect the leash and start the reward. This can be either the aforementioned walk within the park, trip in a car, or whatever else the dog loves to do.

Imparting some kind of reward, whether a treat, a special time out or just a scratch in the back of the ears on every occasion the dog does something you want is an excellent way to keep your dog inspired. If the dog is aware that something remarkable is going to happen whenever it obeys your command, it will be inspired to please you on every occasion.

Puppy/Dogs' Distraction Training

When training any dog, it's far important not to allow distractions disrupt the training. The dog must be trained to disregard distractions, along with different people, different dog, other animals and loud noises, and consequently on what is being taught. These forms of distractions can even be used as rewards when training the dog to return when called.

For example, if your dog enjoys playing with different dogs whether in a local dog park or with the neighbor's dogs, allow it play freely with those other dog. Then move into the park or yard and get in touch with your dog. When it comes to you, provide masses of reward, treats and different rewards, then immediately allow the dog to go out again and play with its friends. Repeat this several times and reward the dog whenever it returns to you. It will quickly understand that coming to you means a great deal (treats and reward) and not bad ones (being taken far from the park).

If the dog does not master this specific kind of training properly, don't get discouraged. Distraction training is one of the hard stuffs to teach. Dogs are obviously social animals, and breaking away from the pack is one of the difficult matters you may ask your dog to do. Most dogs can be understandably reluctant to leave their dog buddies, but it's highly crucial to persist.

Teaching the dog to return to you could require some creativity on your part at the start. For instance, waving a favorite toy, or a treat, is a great way to get your dog's attention and put the focal point back to you. If your dog has been clicker trained, a short click can be a terrific motivator as well.

Once the dog begins to get the grasp of coming when called, you may start to reduce and eliminate the visible cues and attention on getting the dog to respond to your voice on your own. It is crucial that the dog reply to voice commands by itself, in view that you will not usually have in handy toys or other treats as the case may be.

CHAPTER 12

How to Cope with Puppy/Dogs' Separation Tension

Separation tension, additionally regarded to in dog training world as owner absent misbehavior, is one of the more frequently encountered troubles in the world of dog training. Separation tension can occur in lots of extraordinary ways, consisting of chewing, destroying the owner's assets, excessive barking, self-detrimental conduct and careless urination and defecation.

Dog affected by separation anxiety regularly whine, bark, cry, howl, dig, chunk and scratch on the door when the family members are away. Well-meaning owners regularly unsuspectingly inspire this misbehavior through rushing home to reassure the dog, but it's far important for the well-being of each dog and owner that the dog learn how to deal with extended periods of separation.

How the owner leaves the house can often make an impact to separation tension issues. An extended and drawn out period of farewell could make things worse by making the dog feel very lonely when the owner finally leaves. Those lengthy kinds of farewells can get the dog excited, and then leave him with lots of excess power and no way to work it off. These excited, isolated dog regularly work off their extra energy inside the most unfavorable methods, which includes chewing up a favourite rug or piece of furniture.

Extra strength is regularly unsuitable for separation anxiety. If you think that excess amounts of energy may be the problem, try giving your dog more exercises to see if that removes the trouble.

If separation tension is really the trouble, it is vital to cope with the root causes of that anxiety. With the intention to prevent separation tension from occurring, it's far essential for the dog to feel satisfied, safe, and comfortable at the same time as the owner is away for the day. It's far crucial, for example, to give the dog lots of things to keep it busy at the same time as you're away. This means presenting it with lots of toys, including balls or chewing toys. A dog partner is often effective at relieving separation anxiety easily. Giving the dog a playmate, along with some other dog or a cat, is a great way for active owners and pets allike to cope with the strain of being left alone.

Setting apart scheduled play instances, at some stage in which the pet is given your undivided attention, is some other top notch way to alleviate boredom and separation anxiety. Playing with the dog and supplying it with sufficient objects of interest and exercise is a confirmed way to reduce pressure and trauma. A happy dog that has been nicely exercised and properly-conditioned will commonly sleep a day away thankfully and patiently look forward to the return of its owner. It's far critical to set any such day by day play classes earlier before you leave the house every day. It is crucial to calm the dog few minutes after playtime before you go away.

For dog that are already experiencing separation tension and related misbehaviors, it's far important to get them acquainted with your departure. Make certain to practice leaving and returning at abnormal periods, numerous instances during the day. Doing so gets your dog accustomed to your departures and encourages it to understand that you are not leaving him for ever; dog which have been formerly misplaced, or those that have been submitted to shelters and readopted, regularly have the worst problems with separation anxiety. A part of treating this problem is teaching the dog that your leaving isn't always permanent.

Best way to train your dog to not chase people, bicycles, and joggers

Dogs by way of nature are predatory animals, and all predatory animals share the incentive to chase fleeing items. While this is a natural intuition, it isn't always appropriate when those fleeing are joggers, bicyclists or the mailman.

Training the dog not to chase people and bicycles is an essential thing to do, and it's far great to start that training as early as possible. Beginning whilst the dog is still small and non-threatening is important, especially with breeds that develop very big, or with breeds which have popularity for being very competitive. Many people reply to being chased by a dog, especially a massive dog, with understandable fear, and it's great for yourself and your dog that it be trained not to chase earlier before it reaches a threatening extent.

Some dog are simpler to train from chasing than others. Breeds which have been used for watching or herding often control their chasing instincts than different breeds of dogs.

Regardless of what breed of dog you are running with, it's important to not allow it off the leash until its chasing behavior has been curbed. Allowing an untrained dog off the leash is dangerous, irresponsible and illegal.

Before you expose your dog to a state in which it'll

need to chase a person or some thing, be sure to educate it in a safe and controlled enviroment like a fenced backyard. It is important for the dog so that you can keep its focus on you, and for it to understand what conduct you need. The dog should be given the responsibility time and again to carry out the conduct you need while in this controlled setting.

The training session must begin internally within the dog's home. The dog has to be put on a leash and the owner and the dog ought to stand at one end of a hallway or a room. The owner then waves a tennis ball in front of the dog however it doesn't permit it to touch it. After that, the tennis ball is rolled to the other end of the hallway or the room, and the command "stop" is used to tell the dog not to chase the ball. If the dog starts out after the ball, use the command "stop" again and apply a light tug at the leash.

When carrying this sort of training, it's essential that the dog is not allowed to touch the ball. If it reaches the ball, it might imagine that "stop" means to get the ball. This exercise must be repeated numerous times, till the dog has learned the "stop" command. While the dog responds efficiently by not chasing the ball, it should be rewarded with a special treat.

After the dog seems to comprehend this new game, move to another room and try the same thing. Repeat the exercise in several rooms in the house, hall, etc. After the dog has seemingly mastered the training and discovered the use of the "stop" command, you can rehearse with him without the leash; however it is still most effective in a secure vicinity like your private home or a fenced backyard. It is able for the dog to fully manage its chasing instinct, and it's crucial not to hurry the method, or to leave the dog off leash till you're sure it is completely trained.

To check the training, enlist the assistance of a friend to pose as a jogger. It is essential that the dog does not see and recognize this person; it has to assume that it's a stranger in order for the test to be valid. Stand with the dog on its leash and see your buddy jog by multiple times whilst you do the "stop" exercise. If the dog does as it's requested, make sure to provide plenty of reward and treats. If it runs after the "jogger", send a firm reminder via tugging at the leash.

Training your puppy/dog not to chase vehicles

One of the most serious and unusual problematic behaviors among dogs is that of chasing vehicles. Dog ought to understand as early as possible that chasing motors isn't always right. This is because dogs that chase cars in the end become dogs that seize motors, and vehicle plus dog always cause massive trouble.

There are many reasons why dogs chase cars. For one part, chasing shifting items is an ingrained, instinctual conduct that could never be absolutely removed. Chasing behaviors can and must be managed through a number of suitable training and supervision techniques.

A few dogs are extra apt to chase automobiles, bikes, joggers, cats and other dogs than others. Dogs which have a high prey power, along with breeds that have been bred for hunting, are especially susceptible to the thrill of the chase. Herding breeds are also apt to chase vehicles, try to harm the neighbor's youngsters, or express other undesired traits of their breeding.

One reason why most dogs chase cars in particular is that they've found associate vehicles with desirable time and fun things. Most dogs love the experience in the automobile, and after they see a vehicle they may attempt to chase it down for a journey.

Irrespective of what your dog's motivation for chasing cars is, it's far crucial to reduce this risky conduct as quickly as possible.

Training the dog not to chase cars starts with teaching the dog the 'stop' command. The "stop" command is one of the primary tenets of obedience, and it needs to be mastered by each dog.

Coaching the dog to stay where it is, irrespective of the interesting and thrilling matters happening around is very crucial to dog education. In the world of expert dog training, this is known as distraction training. Distraction training may be very essential, and it's far relevant to coaching the dog not to chase vehicles.

Teaching this critical lesson isn't always something you'll be capable of doing on your own. You will need an extra person – a volunteer who will slowly drive by, you may stand with your dog on its leash as the volunteer drives by, having the volunteer drive your own automobile can provide a greater temptation, seeing that dog are in a position to differentiate one vehicle from another. In case your car is the one that the dog often rides in, it's far likely the most tempting item in the world.

While your buddy drives by, either your vehicle or his, watch your dog's response cautiously. If it starts to jump up or pass away, repeat the "stop" command and quickly take your dog back to the sitting position, if it remains where it is, make certain to present it lavish amounts of reward and possibly a treat.

Repeat this procedure for a few days, once your dog is reliably seated when your friend drives by, start lengthening the gap between your self and your dog. A long retractable leash works best. Slowly extend the distance between you and your dogs, ensuring you've got control.

Even after your dog is trained not to chase cars, it is important not to stay out of the leash unsupervised.

Leaving a dog unattended, except inside a nicely and securely fenced environment, is actually asking for problem. Dogs are unpredictable, and it's possible that the chase instinct may want to kick in at precisely the inappropriate moment. The best method is to restrict the dog whilst you can not supervise him.

Training a shy or anxious puppy/dog

With dog as with people, some puppy and dogs are naturally more ambitious and bold than others. While you watch a group of dogs play, it'll quickly end up obvious which one of them is ambitious and which ones are shy. A number of the dog will dangle back at the verge of the pack, perhaps scared of angering the stronger dogs, while others will bounce proper into the fray and begin jostling for control.

Operating with a shy puppy or dog, or one that is anxious, provides its own special challenges. Often ambitious, forceful dogs present tough situations of their own, particularly with control and leadership problems. Every form of dog or puppy has its personal unique traits and its own unique training challenges as a result.

One important reason to build self reassurance in a nervous dog is to save you from biting. Excessive worry dog frequently end up biting to cope with their worry and this sort of fear response can be risky for you and your dog. It is vital to train the dog or puppy that new situations and new human beings are nothing to fear, and that they're not out to harm it.

Symptoms of fear in both dog and dogs consist of being scared of strangers, being leery of new conditions, and averting certain people or gadgets. A nervous domestic dog or puppy can also snap or bite, particularly when cornered.

If you notice signs of worry in your puppy or dog, it's far necessary to act quickly. Fear induced responses can fast turn out to be ingrained in a dog, and as soon as the fear memories are planted they may be hard to erase. Why socializing a younger dog is important to making sure your dog is not apprehensive, and could not grow to be a worry biter. Many dogs are raised as only dog, however even these dogs need to receive the opportunity to play with different dogs and with properly socialized older dogs and friendly cats as well. The more lesson conditions the dog encounters while it's younger, the better it could be able to adapt to new situations as an adult dog.

Adapting to new and changing conditions is a crucial existence ability that each dog need to analyze. As you already know, the world is constantly changing and adapting, and it is crucial that both you and your four legged companion learn to take these adjustments in stride. It's critical for owners to not inadvertently toughen or reward shy or apprehensive behaviors. For example, while a puppy or dog shows worry by whining, crying or hiding, it's natural for the owner to go over and reassure the dog. This form of reassurance can be misinterpreted by the animal as a signal of reward from the pack leader.

While the puppy or dog demonstrates anxious or shy conduct, the excellent method is truly to disregard it. The dog ought to be able to analyze on its own that there is nothing to worry. If left alone, a dog will regularly start to discover the fearful object on its own, thereby getting to know that the initial fear reaction is unsuitable. The owner should permit the dog to discover matters on its own, and not try to cuddle or over guard it.

Another reason for worry reactions, specifically in older dog, is past abuse or lack of right socialization as dogs. The window for good dog socialization is distinctly short, and once this window has closed it is hard to train a dog to socialise with dog and different animals. Likewise, a dog that has been abused in all likelihood has all varieties of bad associations, and it's up to a patient owner to work with the dog to replace those worry reactions with more appropriate responses.

While running with an older anxious dog, it's essential not to attempt to rush the socialization and fear abatement technique. It is best to surely permit the dog to discover things on its very own, even supposing it means it spends a whole lot of time hiding from the perceived monster. Appearing to pressurize the dog to confront the things it fears will do greater damage.

It's also essential to cope with already ingrained fear based total behaviors, which includes biting, snapping and growling, whether or not they resulted from past abuse, a lack of socialization or a mixture of things. If the dog is apprehensive and reacts defensively to strangers, it's important to introduce it slowly. It is critical to correct these risky behaviors and train the dog that fear isn't any excuse for growling, snapping or biting. The best way to do this is to at once reprimand and correct the dog when it bites, snaps or growls at all and sundry.

The dog should be generously rewarded the minute it stops showing aggressive conduct. If you discover yourself reprimanding your dog for displaying competitive behaviors, it is possible you have tried to move him outside too quickly. It's essential to avoid threatening situations an awful lot till the dog has built up the self belief it requires to deal with those conditions. In case you think you have moved too fast, take some steps back and allow the dog regain its confidence.

Coaching your dog to not chew

Chewing is some thing that comes early to each dog. Every dog feels the instinctual need to sharpen its teeth and hone his biting capabilities. Chewing on the right things, like specifically designed chew toys for example, can even help the dog with its teeth and eliminate plaque.

Despite the fact that chewing is natural and healthy, that does not mean that the dog need be allowed to chew everything in sight. It's vital for each dog to learn the difference between the things it's allowed to bite on, like toys and ropes, and the ones which are off limits, together with carpets, footwear and other items.

While working with a new dog, it's far recommended to hold the dog in a small, dog proofed room for a few weeks. This is important to train the dog as well.

Older dogs need to also be constrained to a small place at the start. Doing this lets the dog to slowly acquaint itself to the points of interest in the new family.

While you set up this small, confined region, make sure to provide the puppy or dog with a few proper exceptional chunk toys to keep it entertained while you are not capable of supervising it. Of course the dog should additionally be provided with a warm area to sleep and lots of sparkling easy water.

As the dog is slowly moved to larger portions of the

house, there can be extra opportunities to chunk irrelevant items. Because the dog is given freer access to the home, it is crucial to keep any item that the puppy or dog ought to not chunk, things like rugs, shoes etc, off the ground. If you forget about taking something out and come home to find that the dog has chewed it, fight the urge to punish or yell at the dog. Instead, distract the dog with one of its preferred toys and remove the inappropriate object from its mouth.

The dog ought to then be given one of its favourite toys. Reward the dog when it starts to bite its toy. This will help to train the dog that it gets rewarded if it chews certain objects, but not when it chews other objects.

Teaching the dog what is appropriate to chew is very important, not just for the safety of your high priced furnishings and rugs, but for the protection of the dog in general. Many dogs have chewed risky items like extension cords and so forth. This of course can injure the dog significantly or maybe spark a health problem.

Most dogs examine what to chew and what not to chew quickly, however others are obviously going to be slower than others. Some dogs bite because they're bored, so presenting the dog with plenty of toys and solo activities could be very essential. It is also a very good idea to monitor several play time every day. If the dog is very tired after its play session, possibilities are it can sleep the day away.

Other dog bite to exhibit separation anxiety. Many dog grow to be very nervous when their owners go away, and some dog end up engaged every time the owner is absent. This strain can cause the dog to display all manner of destructive behavior, consisting of chewing or soiling the house. If separation tension is the root of the trouble, the cause of it should be addressed, and the dog confident that you may return.

That is greatly achieved by means of scheduling numerous journeys inside and out of the house every day. At the start, the trips can be just a few minutes, with the duration slowly being extended because the dog's separation tension issues improve.

Educating your dog how not to chunk

Biting is one of the things that every dog seems to do, and each dog must be trained not to do. Like many behaviors, together with leaping up on people, biting and nipping can appear lovable while the domestic dog is small, but a good deal less as it grows older, larger and stronger.

Left to their own toys, most dogs discover ways to control their biting reflex from their mothers and from their littermates. When the doggets over excited when playing the mother dog or the other dog will quickly correct it.

Unfortunately, this type of natural correction often does not arise, on account that many dog are eliminated from their moms whilst they're nevertheless pretty young. It is therefore up to the dog's owner to take over this method.

Socializing the dog with different dogs is one of the satisfactory and most effective approaches to train the dog the ideal and appropriate way to bite, and to curb the biting act. Many communities and pet shops sponsor dog playtime and domestic dog kindergarten lessons, and these training may be fantastic places for dogs to socialize with each other, and with different humans and animals as well. Because the dogs play with different things, they will naturally chew and nip at every thing. While one dog becomes too tough or bites too tough, the other dogs will quick reply by correcting it.

The best time for the socialization of the dog to arise is while it's younger. It's far critical that every dog be well socialized, due to the fact that a poorly socialized dog, or worse, one that isn't socialized at all, can end up dangerous or even neurotic. Most experts recommend that dog be socialized before they have reached the age of 12 weeks, or 3 months.

Some other reasons for socializing the domestic dog early is that mothers of young kids may be understandably reluctant to permit their young children to play with older or large dog. Since socializing the dog with other human beings is just as essential as socializing it with other dog, it's far exceptional to do it when the dog is young enough and is non-threatening to all.

It is essential for the dog to be exposed to a wide range of various stimuli in the course of the socialization method. The socialization technique needed to expose the dog to an extensive form of other animals, consisting of other dogs, adult dog, cats and other domestic animals. In addition, the dog must be placed around humans as possible, together with younger children, older humans, men, women and people from different ethnic backgrounds.

While socialization is important to exposing the dog to various lifestyles, training and preventing it from biting, it isn't always the simplest method of preventing undesirable biting and chewing. Giving the dog suitable things to play with and bite is another way to control the biting. Offering a selection of chunk toys, ropes and other things the dog can chew is crucial to preventing boredom, maintaining its tooth polished and preserving it from chewing things it doesn't have to.

Like all training, it's very important to be steady while teaching the domestic dog not to bite. Each member of the family, in addition to close pals, who can also visit, should all be told that the dog is to be discouraged from biting. If one individual permits the dog to chew on them at the same time as others does not, the dog will quickly turn out to be careless, and that may make the training method a lot more difficult than it should be.

Stopping unwanted urination

Troubles with inappropriate urination are some of the most commonly encountered problems faced by dog owners. Inappropriate urination and defecation is the most commonly stated reason that owners submit their animals to shelters.

Before you can cope with issues with irrelevant urination, it's far essential to recognize the cause of the trouble. There are several reasons why dogs lose control of their bladders, and it is essential to recognize the root cause of the trouble before it can be properly addressed, which include;

Problem #1 – pleasure induced urination

Dog regularly urinate once they appear as overly

excited, and dog which can be otherwise flawlessly controlled every now and then display their pleasure via dripping urine when greeting you excitedly. It's far regular for few dogs to urinate after they get excited, and this could be a particular problem for lots older dogs.

Quite a few pleasure induced urination happens in dog, and it's far due to a loss of bladder control. The dog might not even know it is urinating, and punishment will simply confuse it. Becoming indignant with the dog will quickly cause pleasure induced urination to transform into submissive induced urination, hence compounding the trouble. As the dog grows older and develops higher bladder control, this kind of pleasure induced urination ought to disappear.

The pleasant remedy for pleasure induced urination is prevention. Preventing your dog from becoming over excited is the best way to manage this troubling behavior. In case your dog is worked up via a particular stimulus or scenario, it is important to repeatedly expose it to that state till it no longer causes excessive excitement.

Problem #2 – submissive urination

Submissive urination is a part of pack behavior among animals like dogs and wolves. The submissive member of the pack indicates its submissiveness by lowering itself and urinating. For the reason that dog are pack animals, they'll display their submissiveness to their owner, who they regard as the pack leader by means of displaying this submissive urination.

Dog that exhibit submissive urination are generally displaying their insecurity. Unsocial zed and previously abused dogs regularly show off submissive urination. These dogs want to be seen that there are extra suitable approaches to express their submissive status, together with shaking palms or licking the owner's hand.

The best way to address submissive urination problems is frequently to disregard the urination. Appearing to reassure the dog can provide the wrong effect that you approve of the conduct, while scolding the dog can make the submissive urination worse.

Correcting troubles with submissive urination must be directed at building the dog's self assurance and coaching him in different ways to express his identity. Teaching the dog to lift his paw, take a seat on command, or similar obedience instructions, is a great way to direct the dog's appreciation in an extra suitable way.

Problems with urination are not usually easy to cope with, but it is important to be consistent, and to continually reward suited conduct on the part of the dog. When urination troubles do occur, it's a great idea not to first rule out any clinical situations that would be inflicting the trouble. Scientific problems like bladder infections can be the basic cause of problems with unwanted urination.

After any clinical troubles had been ruled out, it's essential to decide what's inflicting the trouble, and treat it accurately. While it can be tempting to punish the dog for irrelevant urination, doing so will most effectively confuse and similarly intimidate it.

Building self belief and appreciation

The primary thing that any successful animal instructor needs to do is win the confidence and admireation of the animal. This important piece of information absolutely applies to the training of dog. As social pack animals, dogs have a natural need to comply with the leader. Placing yourself as the owner or handler is the idea of any succesful dog training program.

Until your dog has learned to agree and admire you, it will be difficult for any training to be successful. Trust and admiration are not matters that may be compelled, they should be earned through fantastic interaction with your 4 legged associate. After the dog has learned to agree with and admire the owner, you will be surprised at how quickly the training will progress.

Many new dog owners mistake love and affection for trust and appreciation. Even as it is a natural course to bathe your new puppy or dog with love and affection, it is also vital to earn its self assurance and respect. It is also crucial not to allow the domestic puppy or dog to escape with everything it desires to. It is easy to permit a dog take advantage of you, mainly while it's so lovable. It is crucial to set barriers, and to establish ideal and unacceptable behaviors.

Dogs in reality admire those types of boundaries, on account that they are similar to the policies that the pack leader establishes in nature. Each dog inside the pack is aware of what is expected of it, and is aware of its position in the pack order. This kind of established hierarchy allows the pack to hunt and live to tell the tale as a single entity. Your dog is truely searching for this type of management.

If it does not get organization from you, it can get anxious or harassed.

Similarly, failure to earn the honour of the dog may be very bad for the progress of both the human and the dog. A dog that lacks appreciation for its human owner can be dangerous as well as hard to stay with. It's far essential to establish conduct of correction and terrible conduct, and to constantly, effectively enforce the boundaries.

Whilst dealing with a domestic dog, it's very critical to begin gaining its trust and acceptance as quickly as possible. Forming an early bond is the best way to move the training and socialization system forward.

It is also crucial to make the preliminary training periods quick. Dog have a notoriously short interest span, and even older untrained dog can be unable to stay conscious for more than 10 or 15 minutes at a time. It's also satisfactory to make the lesson short and nice than to stretch it out and create a negative mood.

It's also a great idea to begin and close every session with a period of playtime. Beginning and ending the training periods with excessive play is important. Dogs make quick decisions and developing a tremendous affiliation with obedience training will help to create a happy, healthy and nicely-adjusted dog. A happy dog would be less difficult to train, and extra inclined to thrill.

It is also essential to keep the dog from becoming bored all through the training classes. Many dog owners make the mistake of drilling the dog on things like primary obedience talents, heeling, sitting, and so forth. Whilst those obedience skills are crucial, and it's far true that they may form the basis of extra superior abilties, it's important to combine things up and make it a laughing exercise for both your self and your dog. The greater range you provide the better your dog and you will enjoy the training sessions.

CHAPTER 13

Training Your Dog to Disregard Loud Noises

Loud noises, which include fireworks, thunder and site visitors, are one of the most frequently reported by dog owners. It's natural for some dogs to be afraid of loud noises, but few dogs are so traumatized by thunder, fireworks and different loud noises that they're absolutely unable to fathom. Dogs that show excessive fear or phobias can be a risk to themselves and those around them. Dogs may also manifest their worry in self-destructive methods, like slinking underneath the couch or the mattress and getting caught, as an example. They may additionally react in manners which are detrimental to the house, such as urinating or defecating on the carpet, chewing up favorite objects, or barking frequently. Those reactions are often worse while the owner isn't at home. One component that is difficult for many dog owners to comprehend is that soothing or stroking a dog that is displaying worry is exactly the wrong thing to do. Whilst it is natural to try to calm a nervous dog, to the dog you're rewarding it for being afraid. The dog likes the sound of your voice, likes your petting, and concludes that it has accomplished the right thing by acting afraid. This mostly makes a horrifying scenario worse.

The best approach when the dog is expressing worry maybe during a thunderstorm or a fireworks show is to virtually forget about it. It's crucial to observe the dog making sure it does not harm itself, but otherwise simply forget about it and allow it work out the worry on its own. Whilst you go away, make sure there's nothing the dog hide under, for the reason that fireworks or a thunderstorm can pop up at any time.

A dog that is fearful of thunderstorms and other loud noises may additionally need to be restricted to a single room, or even a crate, for a period of time. After the dog feels safe in its "den", it can be capable of addressing its fears a whole better. It could be quite a conflict to teach a dog not to be afraid of thunderstorms, firecrackers and other such noises; however it's critical that the dog at least be capable of managing its fears without being dangerous to itself or its environment.

Using distraction to manage dog fear

Most magicians use show of hands to hide their tricks, so dog owners practice the art of distraction to take their dog's thoughts off their fear. For example, in case your dog is scared of thunderstorms and you recognize one is approaching, collect some of your dog's favorite toys and get prepared for the misdirection.

Of course, your dog will possibly recognise the thunderstorm before you do. When you see your dog begin to display worry, take some of its favorite toys and try to get it to play. Very frightened dogs can be reluctant to play, but it's crucial to try. Frequently a few treats can be a very good distraction. Try shopping for one of those balls that you could fill with treats or biscuits, and encourage your dog to chase it.

Try playing with your dog on every occasion a thunderstorm is in the forecast. This could start to implant good memories, and those can every now and then replace the fear memories that precipitated the dog to be scared of thunderstorms in the first place.

Desensitizing your dog's worry

Desensitization is a particularly powerful way to cope with phobias and fears in humans, and it may be very powerful for dog and other animals as well.

Desensitization entails introducing the dog to small amounts of noises that frighten it. For instance, if the dog is frightened of thunder, try tape recording your subsequent thunderstorm and play it again slowly whilst the dog is comfortable. Reward the dog for not displaying fear responses. If it does display fear responses, do not comfort or soothe it however simply forget about it.

This sort of desensitization training may be remarkably effective for a few dog, but it's going to take lots of patience and tough sessions because the fear of thunder and fireworks aren't always easy to fix.

CHAPTER 14

Solution to Dog Behavioural Problems

Training for correct dog conduct

There are numerous motives for teaching proper dog conduct and coaching, such behavior has many benefits for both the human and dog companions. Dog behavior training is crucial to life and death problems such as preventing aggression, controlling dog on dog aggression problems and coaching dogs to have interaction well with both their handlers and with other members of the circle of relatives.

Information on how dogs advance, and the way dog engage with other animals, is very crucial to understanding how to properly train your dog to be a devoted and dependable associate.

The original dogs were probable orphaned wolf dog followed by early human beings. These wild dog probably learned to act as their human protectors loved, along with guarding the cave or scaring off predators. In exchange for these esteemed behaviors, the people possibly supplied their new partners with food, protection and shelter.

That kind of partnership still exists these days and dogs can still do and perform treasured jobs for its human benefactors. Those jobs consist of herding and guarding farm animals, guarding assets, guarding human beings, and locating games.

Whilst making plans for a dog training program, it's far crucial to recognise that dogs are pack animals.

In wild dog societies, packs are fashioned, and each member of the pack quickly learns its location within the order. Besides, on the occasion of demise or damage to the alpha dog, the hierarchy never changes as soon as it's been mounted. The lower dog understand not to question the alpha dog, and the alpha dog understands his location as leader of the pack.

All of the different dogs within the pack look to the alpha dog for leadership in critical cases like locating food and keeping off large predators. So to educate your dog and cement your position, it is vital for it to recognise you to be the alpha dog.

This is because a dog that sees its owner as a superior leader will comply with the instructions the owner offers without question. Getting the respect of the dog is the most crucial step to proper dog training, and it's going to form the basis of all subsequent training.

The motives for training a dog properly are many, particularly in today's society. A nicely-mannered, obedient dog is a pleasure to be around, both for the owner and his or her family, and for humans in the society at large. Furthermore, seeing a nicely-mannered dog sets human beings's mind comfortably, in particular breeds which are perceived to be dangerous, which include dobermans, rottweilers and pit bulls.

When training dog and managing unwanted dog behaviors, it's vital to understand the motivating factors behind those behaviors. For instance, many dog showcase unwanted behaviors associated with chewing and destroying fixtures due to separation tension. Handling the causes of these behaviors is a critical first step to eliminating those problematic behaviors.

Many dog exhibit undesirable behaviors as a result of pressure within the animal's lifestyles, and its incapability to deal with that pressure. The purpose of an amazing dog training program is to allow the dog to endure extra levels of strain without turning into a problematic animal.

Whilst managing dog conduct, it is essential not to confuse human conduct with dog conduct. Even as there may be temptations on the part of dog owners to see their dogs as nearly human, in fact dog and humans have very specific drives, and one of a kind reaction to comparable conditions.

One trait that human beings and dogs do share is the need to shape the social groups and bond within social companies. This bonding is important to both humans and dog, as both species have developed and changed over time.

Dog training for favored behaviors

Teaching a dog proper conduct when it is younger could be very critical. Even as playing and having an exciting time with your new dog or puppy is without a doubt important, it's also critical to train your dog accordingly to what's expected, which behaviors are suited and which behaviors aren't perfect.

Teaching those lessons early, whilst the dog is still a puppy, is a pleasant guarantee that these lessons may be retained. Dog understand quickly, and each interaction between human and dog is teaching the dog something. Making sure you're teaching the proper training is important to you because you are the dog handler.

Right education strategies are important for the safety of the dog in addition to the protection of the family and the commuity at large. Whilst dog are loving, protective participants of the circle of friends in most instances, a poorly trained dog can be dangerous and detrimental. Making sure your new addition is a pleasure to be around and not a threat is satisfying to the owner.

The connection among human beings and dogs dates as far back as hundreds of years, and dogs were domesticated longer than any other animals. Therefore, human beings and dogs have formed a bond not shared among other domesticated animals. This strong bond could be very useful while training any dog.

All dog owners and dog trainers should understand how dog society works within the absence of people. It's far vital to recognize the pack hierarchy, and to use that hierarchy to your benefit as you train your dog. All pack animals have a lead animal, in the case of dogs it is the alpha dog. All contributors of the pack look to the alpha dog for direction and steerage. The alpha dog makes crucial organization in searching, averting other predators, protecting territory and other important survival skills. This pack arrangement is what has allowed wolves and wild dog to be such successful predators, while other big predators have been driven to extinction.

What all this means to you as the dog instructor is that you ought to set your self up as the pack leader, the alpha dog if you will – so you can earn the respect and trust of your dog. If the dog does not see you as its superior and its leader, you will not get very far in your training.

Admiration isn't something that can be forced. It's

something that is earned through the interaction of humans and dog. As the dog learns to admire and contemplate you, you will start to make amazing strides in your training program. Training based on mutual appreciation and trust is much more likely to prevail ultimately than one that is based totally on worry and intimidation.

A fearful dog is prone to becoming a biting dog, and that is sincerely one thing you do not need in your house. Rewarding the dog while it does the right thing, in preference to punishing it for doing the wrong thing, is crucial to the fulfillment of any training program.

Punishment confuses and similarly frightens the

dog, and it may set the training course weeks back if not months. It is vital to provide the dog the choice to do the proper thing or the wrong thing, and to reward the dog when it makes the right choice. For example, if the dog chases joggers, have a friend jog by while you keep the dog on the leash. If the dog attempts to chase the "jogger", take a step and backtrack it, then start once more. You aren't punishing this wrong decision; you're sincerely providing the solution. While the dog sits flippantly through your side, deliver it a treat and lots of reward. The dog will quickly examine that sitting is the right choice and chasing the jogger is the wrong one.

Removing biting behaviors

Bringing home a brand new dog is constantly an interesting time. Introducing the new dog to the family needs to be an exciting time for both you and your dog. One of the first challenges, however, to the excitement of the new dog, is curtailing umpleasant dog behaviors.

Stop biting and mouthing

Biting and mouthing is a common pastime for many dog and puppies. Dogs evidently chunk and mouth each other whilst playing with siblings, and they amplify this behavior to their human partners. While other dogs have thick skin, however, human beings do not, so it's essential to educate your domestic dog on what is suitable, and what is not on the subject of the use of those sharp enamel.

The first part of training the domestic dog is to inhibit the biting reflex. Biting might be adorable and harmless with a five pound dog, however it's neither adorable nor innocent when that dog has grown to adulthood. Consequently, dogs have to learn to manipulate their bite earlier before they attain the age of four (4) months. Dog usually discover ways to inhibit their chunk from their moms and their littermates, but considering the fact that they may be taken away from their moms while young, many never understand this crucial lesson. It is therefore up to the people within the dog's existence to teach this lesson.

One remarkable way to inhibit the biting reflex is to permit the dog to play and socialize with other dog and socialized older dogs. Dog love to tumble, roll and play with each other, and whilst dog play they chew differently constantly. This is the satisfactory manner for dogs to discover ways to manage themselves when they chew. If one dog will become too difficult when playing, the rest of the pack will punish him for that behavior. Through this kind of socialization, the dog will learn to control its biting reflex.

Proper socialization has other blessings as well, including teaching the dog not to be frightened of other dogs. Dog which might be allowed to play with different dog, study important socialization capabilities, commonly discover ways to become better members in their human family. Dog that get less socialized can be more unfavorable, more hyperactive and display other troubling behaviors. Furthermore, lack of socialization in dogs regularly causes fearful and competitive behaviors to widen. Dog frequently react aggressively to new conditions, especially if they're not well socialized. In order for a dog to grow to be a member of the community in addition to the family, it must be socialized with different humans, especially kids. Dogs make a distinction between their owners and other people, and between children and adults. It's far essential, therefore, to introduce the dog to both kids and adults.

The best time to socialise a dog with young kids is while it is nonetheless very young, generally while it is 4 months old or young. One motive for this is that mothers of young kids can be understandably reluctant to allow their youngsters play with huge dog or older dogs. That is especially correct with massive breed dogs, or with breeds of dog that have a reputation for competitive conduct.

How to use Trust to save you from being bitten

Teaching your house dog to trust and appreciate you is a completely effective way to prevent biting. Gaining the trust and respect of your dog is ideal for all dog training, and for correcting troublesome behaviors.

It is crucial to in no way hit or slap the dog, both throughout training or any other time. Physical punishment is the most suitable way to erode the progress of an effective education program. Reprimanding a dog will not prevent him from biting, it will truly scare and confuse him.

Training a domestic dog not to chunk is an important part of any dog education training. Biting behaviors that are not corrected will best worsen, and what appeared like innocent behavior in a dog can fast expand to risky, detrimental behavior in an adult dog.

Everybody who owns a dog or dog will sooner or

later run into the need to eliminate unwanted habits. While most dogs are eager to thrill their owners and clever enough to do what is requested of them, it is important for the owner to properly say just what constitutes desirable and unacceptable behaviors.

Each sort of unacceptable behavior calls for its own personal particular treatments, and in most instances the healing procedures will need to be tailor-made to fit the unique personality of the dog. Each breed of dog has its very own specific personality characteristics, and each person inside that breed has his or her very own precise personality.

How to solve chewing problem

Dogs obviously bite, and they have a tendency to explore the use of their mouths and teeth. Whilst chewing can be regular, however, it isn't desirable, and it's far vital to nip any chewing issues within the bud to save the chewing dog from developing right into a chewing dog.

Supplying a selection of chunk toys is important whilst coaching a domestic dog what's suitable to bite and what is not. Offering a variety of appealing chew toys is a good manner to keep the domestic dog entertained and to keep his tooth and gums exercised. Scented or flavored toys are best picks for most dog.

The dog ought to be endorsed to play with those chosen toys, and the domestic dog ought to be effusively rewardd on every occasion it plays with or chews these toys.

Some other terrific method is to encourage the dog to pick a toy on every occasion it greets you. Whenever the dog greets you or a member of your own family, teach it to get a toy among its favourite toys.

It's also crucial to workout top housework strategies when training a dog to not chunk on objects. Keeping the location to which the domestic dog has access. Keeping gadgets out of reach of the dog will go a long way towards discouraging irrelevant chewing. Attempt to keep the dog's location free of shoes, trash, and different objects, and always make certain that the region has been properly dog proofed.

If the dog does pick up an inappropriate item like a shoe, distract the dog and quickly replace the item with one of its toys. After the dog has taken the toy, reward it for playing with and chewing that toy.

Eliminating hassle behaviors while training your domestic dog. Sadly, getting rid of worrisome behaviors is one issue that most dog owners in the end face. This part of this book will identify some of the most encountered behaviorial issues;

Problem #1 – leaping up on people

One of the most common issues often referred to

with dogs is that of jumping up on people. Alas, that is one of those behaviors which might be frequently inadvertently encouraged by owners. After all, it's far lovely and adorable when that little 10 pound dog jumps up on you, your own family members and your pals. Many humans reward this conduct on the part of a small dog with kisses and treats.

This is a huge mistake; however, when you consider that, your adorable little dog may soon grow to be a complete grown up dog who could weigh a hundred kilos, that jumping behavior is not quite so lovely, likewise to being annoying, leaping up on humans may be dangerous. A massive, heavy dog, jumping enthusiastically, can effortlessly knock over a toddler or an older or handicapped adult. In today's controversial society, such an incident ought to easily scare you, because it leaves the dog's owner with the problem of an undesirable lawsuit.

The time to train a dog that is jumping up on humans while it's still young is clean to handle. Retraining a dog that has been allowed to leap up on human beings may be difficult for the owner, and complicated for the dog.

Whilst the doggy tries to leap on you or every other member of your own family, gently but firmly place the dog's lower back to the floor. After the dog is standing firmly at the ground, be sure to reward it.

It is critical for each member of the family, as well as regular pals, to take in this rule and observe it meticulously. If one member of the family reprimands the dog for leaping and another rewards it, the dog will be understandably confused. As with other dog training issues, consistency is the key to coaching the dog that jumping is beside the point.

While praising the dog for staying down, it is crucial for the teacher to get down on the dog's level. Giving affection and reward at eye stage with the dog is a tremendous way to reinforce the lesson.

Problem #2 – pulling and tugging at the leash

Pulling on the leash is another problematic trait that many dogs pick up. Alas, this behavior is one that is now and again encouraged by well-meaning owners.

Playing games like tug of war with the leash, or maybe with a rope (which can look like the leash to the dog) can unwittingly encourage a problematic conduct.

The use of a best frame handle may be a huge help when training a dog to not pull, or retraining a dog that has picked up the dependancy of pulling on the leash. Try training the dog to simply accept the frame with the same manner it accepts the everyday buckle collar.

While strolling with your dog, try using a toy to inspire the dog to remain at your side. A training collar well used, can also be an excellent education tool for a troublesome dog. While using a training collar or choke chain, however, it is very essential to fit correctly, and to use a rope that is neither too massive nor too small for your dog.

While walking along with your dog, it's far vital to hold the leash free at all times. If the dog starts to tug in advance, the handler needs to instruct the dog quickly. It is important to use a short tug, observed by means of an instantaneous slackening of the leash. When training a dog, it's far essential to never let the dog pull you around. Training the dog to walk well is certainly vital, especially while coping with a large breed of dog. If your hundred and fifty pound extraordinary dog hasn't found out how to stroll well even if it remains a 20 pound dog, possibilities are, it will in no way learn.

It is crucial to yank or pull on the dog's neck whilst correcting him. A mild, constant strain will work tons better than a difficult yank. The acceptable strategy is to apply the least amount of strain neccesary to acquire the preferred end result.

Problem #3 - escaping and roaming the neighborhood

A responsible dog owner could in no way dream of allowing his or her dog to roam the neighborhood freely. Allowing a dog to roam on its own is irresponsible, dangerous (to the dog and the neighborhood), and likely even unlawful. Most towns have ordinances which limit dog from being allowed to roam round loose, so you might be at risk of imprisonment if your dog is found wandering the community unjustly.

Of course occasionally, the wandering dog isn't always the owner's idea, and lots of dogs carry out feats of getting away when left on their own. The temptations for unattended dogs are many, such as passing bicycles, joggers, kids, cats and different dogs. It's a great deal easier to stop a dog from escaping than to recapture an unfastened dog, eliminating the inducement to escape is a massive part of the solution. A bored dog is more likely to spend its day plotting a top notch escape. A dog that is surrounded with masses of toys, a smooth bed, and masses of sparkling clean, water, is more likely to spend its day contentedly napping or playing with toys till the owner returns.

Similarly, a dog with plenty of pent up, unused power will likely try and escape. Try to incorporate several vigorous play sessions with your dog into your daily activities. Make one of these play classes earlier than you leave. It is also essential to make the opportunities of a break out as dim as possible, through proper fencing and different measures. For dog that dig, it may be important to extend the fence underground with the aid of putting metallic stakes in the floor every few feet. For dogs that bounce, it may be necessary to make the fence higher. And if none of these measures work, it may be essential to confine the dog to the house while you are not at home.

How to handle excess whining, howling and immoderate barking

Start with one of the most frequently encountered problematic behaviors in both dog and puppies. While a few barking and different vocalizing is perfectly regular, in many cases barking, howling and whining can turn out to be complicated. That is specifically crucial for the ones residing in rental buildings, or in closely spaced houses. Fielding court cases about barking isn't always the excellent way for you and your dog to meet the buddies.

A few recommendations of handling excessive whining, barking and howling are:

✓ In case your puppy or dog is howling or whining while restrained to its crate, straight away take it to its rest room region. Most dog and puppiess will whine when they need to do their shitty business.It's very essential to train a dog or a dog to accept being on its own. Many dog suffer from separation anxiety, and these worried dog can exhibit all types of negative and annoying behaviors. It's far important to familiarize the dog to being left on its own, even if the owner is at home.

✓ Constantly strive to make the house puppy or dog at ease as possible. Constantly attend to the bodily and psychological desires of the dog via meals, water and toys.

✓ If the dog is whining, check for obvious reasons first. Is the water dish empty? Is the dog displaying signs and symptoms of contamination? Has its favourite toy rolled below the fixtures? Is the temperature of the room too hot or too bloodless?

✓ Do not reward the dog or puppy for whining. If the dog whines whilst left alone, as an instance, it'd be a mistake to visit the dog whenever it whines.

✓ After you have ensured that the dog's physical desires are being met, and that pain is not responsible for the whining, do not hesitate to reprimand the dog for irrelevant behavior.

Refusing to come when called

Many dog owners fail to apprehend the importance of getting a dog to come when called until there's trouble, both with the collar or leash breaking, or the dog breaking free to chase someone or every other animals. These situations can be dangerous for the dog, the owner and other members of the community. In regions where there is a lot of vehicular traffic, the situation may even be deadly to the dog.

Unfortunately, many owners sabotage this crucial part of their dog's education by way of permitting it to run off leash and unattended to. Whether or not the dog is authorized to run inside the park, at the seaside, or just play with other dog, this teaches the dog that there are numerous things that do not involve its owner. In truth, from the dog's perspective, those fun instances are frequently ruined by the appearance of the owner.

Observe instances from the dog's attitude for a moment. You and the dog are having a tonne of excitement going for walks on the seashore with all of your dog buddies, and all at once here comes this human to take you faraway from the fun. When you see the dog's point of view it is simple to see how the appearance of the owner and the leash may be understood.

This negative notion causes many dogs to delay this outcome by refusing to come when called. From the dog's point of view, the dog has learned that the most rewarding thing to do is to ignore the call of its owner. At the same time as this will appear like a good idea to the dog, it is no longer a great issue from the owner's perspective.

For dog who have not yet found out this kind of avoidance behavior, it is satisfying to save yourself from this dilemma by supervising the dog at play, and making the time you spend with your dog as plenty, or more, amusing, as the time it spends alone with other dogs. For dog which have already learned the act of ignoring their owner, some retraining is paramount. It's far important that the dog reply to the *"come here"* command, for the protection of both people and dog itself.

One factor to keep away from, is following the *"come here"* command with unpleasant activities like calling the dog and then without delay giving him a bathtub, clipping his nails, taking him to the vet, and so forth. This will fast teach the dog that coming to the owner has terrible consequences. It is crucial to ask the dog to come after which you play, feed, stroll with it or interact in other fun activities. In case you do want to take your dog to the vet, shower it, etc. Be sure to give it some time so the dog does not associate the *"come here"* command with the awful activities.

It is essential to understand that dogs are continuously getting to know, whether or not a formal training session is on or not. Your dog is constantly learning something from you, whether correct or dreadful. It's therefore vital to make each interaction with your dog a fantastic one. While training the dog to come on command, it's crucial that the dog be constantly rewarded every time it does as the owner commands. A reward may be as easy as a pat on the head, or a scratch at the back of the ears. Of course, treats with rewards are loved, and lots of dog are surprisingly inspired by food and reply quickly to this kind of training. The secret is to be consistent. The dog has to get some kind of reward, whether it is reward, a toy, or a treat every time it acts in accordance with the owner's wishes.

Conclusion

The idea of training any animal is fundamentally to getting it to agree with you, having confidence and earning your respect. Genuine training can't begin till the animal has identified you as its leader and admire you and entrusted you with its confidence.

The error many dog owners make is mistaking love and affection for recognition and self assurance. While it's very crucial to like your new dog, it's also very crucial that the dog recognizes you and notices you as his leader. Dog are certainly pack animals, and every dog looks to the lead dog for recommendation and direction. Making you the pack leader is essential to the success of training any dog.

Failure to gain the honour of the dog can create a disobedient, out of control and even risky dog. Difficult dog are dangerous, whether or not they may be created through awful breeding, owner ignorance or wrong training. It's far vital to train the dog right from the start, for the reason that retraining a troublesome dog is a lot difficult than training a dog properly for the first time.

It's very important for any new dog owner, whether or not operating with a 12 weeks old dog or a twelve years old dog, to at once get the honour of the animal. That doesn't suggest the use of difficult or risky managing methods, however it does mean letting the dog know that you are in control of the state of affairs. Dogs want structure in their lives, and they'll not resent the owner for taking control. As a member of the pack, the dog will recognize your taking the position of teacher and coach as you start your training session.

When operating with the dog, it's far essential to keep the training classes short before everything. This is especially crucial when operating with a younger dog, since puppies have a tendency to have an awful lot shorter interest span than older dog, keeping the training session quick, and fun, is crucial for proper education.

When starting the training session, you need to be

conscious of the most basic instructions. The heel command is one of the fundamental, and one of the simplest to teach. Start by putting the puppy or dog in a properly geared up training collar. Be sure to follow the instructions for fitting and sizing the shade to ensure that it really works as planned.

Begin to walk and allow your dog to stroll beside you. If the dog charges off, lightly pull the leash. This in turn will tighten the training collar and correct the dog. If the gentle strain is ineffective, it can be important to slowly increase pressure. Constantly be cautious to not over-correct the dog. The use of an excessive amount of pressure may want to frighten the dog and scare it further. If on the otherhand, the dog lags behind, the owner need to lightly encourage it till it is walking beside the owner.

Most dog carry out the heeling idea pretty hastily, and quickly learn that they have to stroll beside their owners, neither lagging behind nor pulling ahead. As soon as the dog has mastered heeling at a moderate tempo, the owner needs to slow his or her pace and allow the dog to modify along with it. The owner has to additionally accelerate the tempo and allow the dog to hurry up as well. In the end, strolling frequently will beef up the lesson that the dog should always walk at the heel of the handler.

From heeling, the subsequent step must be to halt on command. This halt command works properly as an accessory to heel. As you're walking, stop and watch your dog. Many dog without delay comprehend that they're anticipated to stop when their handler does. Others can also need the reminder of the leash and the training collar.

After the halt on command has been mastered, the handler needs to encourage the dog to sit on command as well. Once the dog has stopped, the handler lightly pushes on the dog's hindquarters to encourage it to sit down. Usually, after this walk, halt, sit procedure has been achieved a few instances; the dog will start to sit on its own whenever it stops. Of course, it's important to offer outstanding reward, and possibly even a treat, every time the dog does as it's expected.

In conclusion, if you've accompanied all the courses in this book carefully you must be geared up to begin training your puppy/dog with the most complex hints and behaviors listed in this book. Always remember to be patient and constantly use high-quality reinforcement to educate your dog.

Dog which are abused or scared into obedience regularly don't have an actual knowledge of the actions they understand and express different behavioral problems that might make them a risk to you or your circle of friends. With a little persistence and lots of love, you and your dog friend can be enjoying each other's companionship without stress or behavioral issues at all times!

About the Author

Micah Jack is a dog trainer with modern and friendly approach for bringing out the best in all varieties of dog breed. Jack helps you tailor training to your dog's unique traits and energy level; leading to quicker results and a much happier pet.